Disclaimer

MW01598842

Medicine and nursing are conti.. believed to be reliable and accurate and have made every effort to provide information that is up to date with best practices at the time of publication. Despite our best efforts we cannot disregard the possibility of human error and continual changes in best practices the author, publisher, and any other party involved in the production of this work can warrant that the information contained herein is complete or fully accurate. The author, publisher, and all other parties involved in this work disclaim all responsibility from any errors contained within this work and from the results from the use of this information. Readers are encouraged to check all information in this book with institutional guidelines, other sources, and up to date information. For up to date disclaimer information please visit: http://www.nrsng.com/about.

NCLEX®, NCLEX®-RN ®are registered trademarks of the National Council of State Boards of Nursing, INC. and hold no affiliation or support of this product.

Photo Credits:
All photos are original photos taken or created by the author or rights purchased at Fotolia.com. All rights to appear in this book have been secured.

Some images within this book are either royalty-free images, used under license from their respective copyright holders, or images that are in the public domain. Images used under a creative commons license are duly attributed, and include a link to the relevant license, as per the author's instructions. All Creative Commons images used under the following license. All works in the public domain are considered public domain given life of the author plus 70 years or more as required by United States law.

1

Fluids, Electrolytes and Acid Base Balance

for Nurses

NRSNG.com | NursingStudentBooks.com

Jon Haws RN CCRN

Sandra Haws RD CNSC

©TazKai LLC 2015

Your Free Gift!
As a way of saying thanks for your purchase, I'm offering a
free PDF download:

"63 Must Know NCLEX® Labs"

With these charts you will be able to take the 63 most
important labs with you anywhere you go!
You can download the 4 page PDF document by clicking here,
or going to NRSNG.com/labs

Contents

Fluid and Electrolyte Basics

Fluids and electrolytes play a vital role in homeostasis within the body by regulating various bodily functions including cardiac, neuro, oxygen delivery and acid-base balance and much more.

Electrolytes are the engine behind cellular function and maintain voltages across cellular membranes. Without proper electrolyte balance the body is unable to carry out the most basic functions.

Understanding the basics of these complex concepts is vital to your success in caring for complex patients.

This book covers the essentials of fluids, electrolytes and acid-base balance. Toward the end of the book you will find case studies, charts, graphs, cheat sheets, and 43 NCLEX style questions covering fluids and electrolytes.

Movement of Fluids and Electrolytes

Movement of Fluid

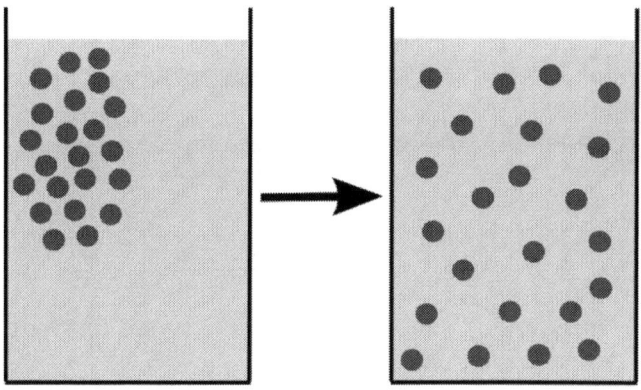

Concentration

Concentration is a number that shows the amount of solutes dissolved in a fluid. The word solute is used to describe any substance that is dissolved in a fluid.

Concentration gradient: Molecules in a solution are in a constant state of motion. In a liquid, they will naturally move from areas of higher concentration to areas of lower concentration. A concentration gradient is simply variations in concentrations in a fluid. In the following picture the container on the left has an area to the upper left that has higher concentration than the rest of the container.

Osmolarity: The number of particles in a solution by volume (mOsm/L). It is calculated using osmolality.

Osmolality: The number of particles in a solution by mass (mOsm/kg). This can be measured using an osmometer. Osmolality is used- more so than osmolarity- in a clinical setting. The osmolality of IV fluids, plasma, urine are used to help paint a picture of volume status in a patient. Osmolality creates osmotic pressure and thus affects movement of water from different compartments in the body.

Pressure

Pressure is a force applied to a surface. Different forces affect movement of water through different areas of the body.

Osmotic Pressure: Pressure needed to stop fluid movement across a membrane created by concentration gradients. When molecules can't move across a membrane, fluid will move to equilibrate the concentrations.

Oncotic pressure: A type of osmotic pressure. It is specifically talking about the pressure needed to stop movement of fluid in response to protein concentrations. Albumin in the blood creates oncotic pressure that helps keep blood within the vessels of the circulatory system.

Hydrostatic pressure: Pressure created by the pull of gravity. Hydrostatic pressure can also be created by blood against the surface of our vessels. Blood pressure created by the heart pumping is hydrostatic pressure.

Movement

Osmosis: Osmosis is the movement of fluid across a membrane due to a concentration gradient.

Filtration: Filtration occurs when water moves across a membrane due to hydrostatic pressure. An example would be pouring a solution through a colander. The force of gravity aids in the movement of the fluid.

Tonicity

When we talk about tonicity we are comparing two different solutions. Tonicity is a term to describe the effect of the particles in concentration on osmolality. If a particle is small and can pass through the membrane it will have little effect on osmolality, because the concentration can even out by movement of the particle instead of the fluid. All body fluids have equal tonicity, because fluids will move between compartments to balance things out. In medicine we are typically comparing the tonicity of different IV fluids to the blood. If we add an IV fluid and change the blood concentration that can effect water movement between plasma and the inside of red blood cells.

Hypertonic: A hypertonic solution has a higher concentration than blood. There are more solutes dissolved in the solution.

Isotonic: An isotonic solution has the same concentration as blood.

Hypotonic: A hypotonic solution has a lower concentration of fluid than the blood.

Hypertonic	Isotonic	Hypotonic

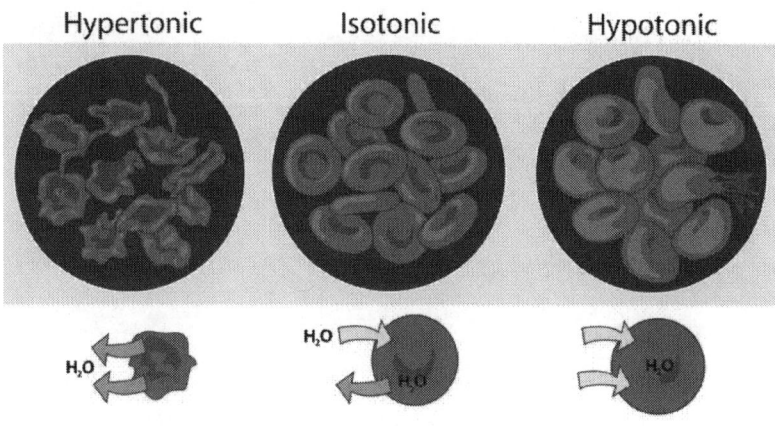

Movement of Electrolytes

Some particles in the body can move through membranes easily, while others may need to be transported or assisted with a little pressure. In this section we will discuss different types of movement that occur across body **membranes**.

Membranes

Different areas of the body are separated by different types of membranes:

Cell membranes: The cell membrane separates cells from the outside environment, intracellular fluid from interstitial or intravascular fluid.

Capillary membranes: The walls of the blood vessels. They separate intravascular fluid from interstitial fluid.

Epithelial membranes: Mucosa of the stomach, intestines, and renal tubules.

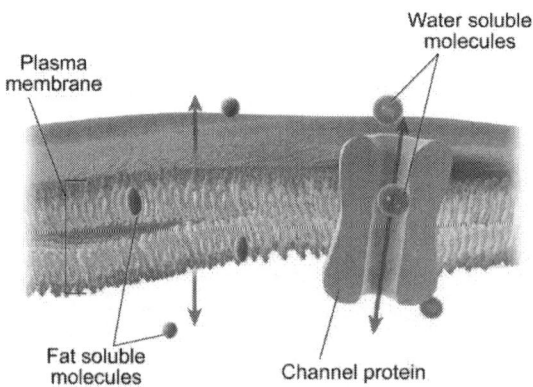

Diffusion Across the Plasma Membrane

The cell membrane contains two layers of phospholipids which have a hydrophilic head (tendency to mix with water) and hydrophobic tail (repelled from water). The hydrophilic tails point toward each other with the hydrophobic heads line each side of the membrane. Embedded in the membranes are different proteins. Because of the nature of the membrane some particles can move freely while others must be transported.

Diffusion: Diffusion occurs when solutes in a solution move from an area of higher concentration to an area of lower concentration. There must be a concentration gradient for diffusion to occur. Diffusion in the body is affected by several different factors: **temperature, concentration, size of molecule, and surface area of membrane.** Diffusion may also occur due to an electrical gradient. If positively charged ions move into the cell they will be followed by negatively charged ions.

Simple diffusion: Simple diffusion occurs when substances are lipid soluble (oxygen, carbon dioxide) or when they are small enough to travel through protein pores or channels (urea, water). Simple diffusion requires a concentration or electrical gradient.

Facilitated diffusion: Large molecules or molecules that aren't lipid soluble require facilitated diffusion. Concentration gradients need to be present in facilitated diffusion. Because of its size glucose requires a **carrier protein**, which allows it to become lipid soluble to move through the cell membrane. Carrier proteins can become saturated if there is a very large difference in concentration between the inside of the cell and the outside.

Active transport: Active transport is required to move molecules against a concentration or chemical gradient. Energy is required for active transport to take place. The sodium-potassium pump is an example of active transport. Carrier proteins can become saturated with excess substrate (molecule upon which an enzyme acts).

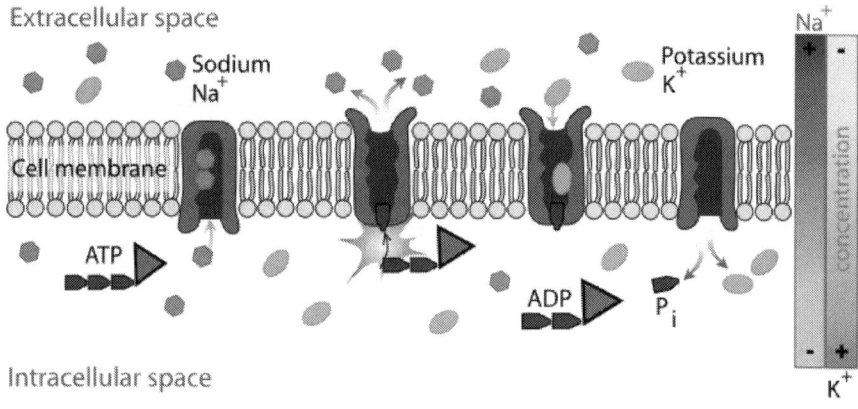

To put everything together, the body has many different compartments. Fluids found in each compartment are regulated by membranes, concentrations, and hydrostatic pressure.

Water can move freely from vessels into cells or interstitial spaces. The pressures described above help maintain fluids within the different compartments. The next section describes each of the different areas where fluid is kept and how the different regulatory mechanisms help maintain homeostasis.

Fluids in the Body

The body is made of trillions of cells. Water is found around cells, inside cells, within vessels, and around organs. Each fluid in the body has unique characteristics that allow for the specific functions within each space. The body has many regulatory mechanisms to maintain homeostasis of the fluids.

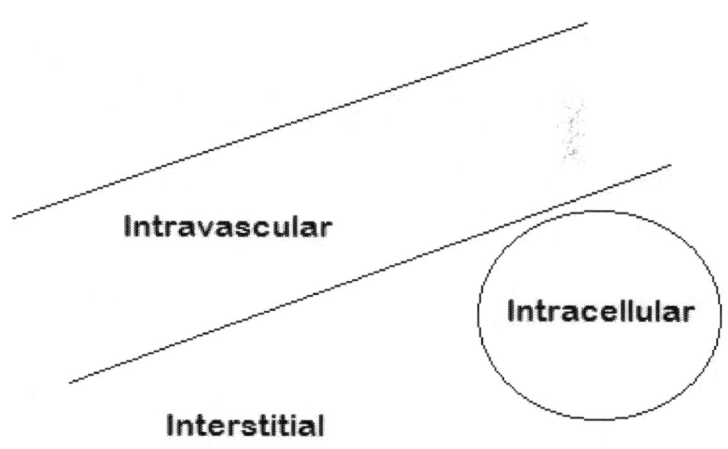

Total body water: 40 liters

Extracellular fluid: Fluid outside of the cell. ECF includes fluids within the blood vessels (intravascular fluid) and fluid within the interstitial spaces. ECF totals about **15 Liters**.

Intravascular Fluid: This includes all the blood within the circulatory system: veins

15

and arteries. IVF, also known as blood contains red blood cells and Plasma. The plasma makes up 3 liters out of 5 liters of IVF.

Interstitial Fluid: Interstitials fluid is found in many compartments throughout the body. Some examples include lymph, synovial fluid, cerebrospinal fluid, digestive secretions, and pericardial fluid. **11-12 liters of fluid**.

Intracellular fluid: The fluid components within the cell are the cytoplasm and neoplasm. Intracellular fluids make up 60% of total body water. **25 liters.**

The different fluids in the body are unique in their electrolyte content. The following chart lists the electrolyte content of different fluids in the body and compares them to the IV fluid that most resembles plasma: lactated ringers.

	Na+	K+	Ca+	Mg+	HCO_3^-	Cl^-
Plasma	142	5	5	2	26	102
Interstitial fluid	144	4			30	114
Intracellular fluid	10	160			8	2
Lactated Ringers	130	4	3		28	109

Fluid Balance

Fluid Gain		Fluid Loss	
Metabolism	300 mL	Urine	1200-1500 mL
Beverages	1100-1400 mL	Skin	500-600 mL
Food	800-1000 mL	Lungs	400 mL
		GI Tract	100-200 mL
Total	**2200-2700 mL**	**Total**	**2200-2700 mL**

Fluid Gain

Fluids are added to the body in the following ways.

Metabolism

When carbohydrates, proteins, and fats are broken down water is released in the process. It is not a huge contributor but does provide about **300 mL water daily**.

Beverages

How much we drink may vary quite a bit day to day. The body controls water intake to some extent by stimulating thirst. All beverages contain water and we absorb water based on demand. Typically water intake is **1100-1400 mL/day**, but this can be drastically higher during times of extreme water loss (diabetes, hot environment, extreme exercise, etc.)

Food

Many foods in our diet have a good water content. Some of the biggest contributors are soups and fruits. The amount varies with the amount and type of food, but generally provides about **800-1000 mL water per day**.

Fluid Loss

Fluids are lost from the body in the following ways.

Urine

The kidneys filter 180 Liters of plasma each day. The kidneys typically produce between **1200-1500 mL of urine daily**, and can concentrate urine between 50- 1200 mOsm/kg. However, urine is typically between 300-900 mOsm/kg. The concentration is determined by available water or the amount of waste that needs to be excreted. If the blood volume is low the kidneys will produce concentrate urine that is low in sodium. To remove a typical day's waste the kidneys need to produce a **minimum of 400 mL of urine**.

Three common terms are used to describe urine production:

    oliguria: < 400 mL urine in 24 hours
    anuria: < 100 mL urine in 24 hours
    polyuria: increased urine output

Skin

Insensible fluid loss: Water loss via the skin. This occurs due to diffusion, and it is **pure water** (no solute).

Sensible fluid loss: This is also known as sweat and contains water and electrolytes. In extreme cases we can lose up to 2 liters/hour of extra fluid.

Lungs

When we breathe our body humidifies the air and water is lost in the air that we breathe out. We lose about **400 mL per day** via breathing. This is also classified as an **insensible loss.**

GI Loss

We typically only lose **100-200 mL per day** via the GI tract, however when things go wrong we can lose a lot more. Each day 3-6 liters are secreted into the GI tract and reabsorbed, that is about 1/3 of total ECF fluid. In cases of nasogastric tube suction, vomiting, or diarrhea significant fluids can be lost.

Stomach: isotonic fluid with Na+, K+, Cl⁻ , H+
Small intestines: isotonic fluid with Na+, K+, bicarbonate (HCO3)
Large intestines: hypotonic fluids

Third-space fluid shifts

Third-space fluid shifts are shifts of water **from intravascular space to interstitial space**. When this happens a patient will look fluid overloaded but will also shows signs of volume depletion with hypotension and tachycardia. The following are examples of third-space fluid shifts:

Ascites: fluid movement into the peritoneal cavity because of cirrhosis or hepatic venous obstruction

Peritonitis: fluid movement into the peritoneal cavity

Small bowel obstruction: fluids are secreted into the small intestines and reabsorbed in the large intestines. When an obstruction occurs the fluid remains in the small bowel.

Burns: fluid movement into interstitial space due to increased capillary permeability and decreased vascular osmotic pressure.

In third-space fluid shifts the fluid is **not available** to the cells or the intravascular space.

Kidney's Role in Fluid and Electrolyte Balance

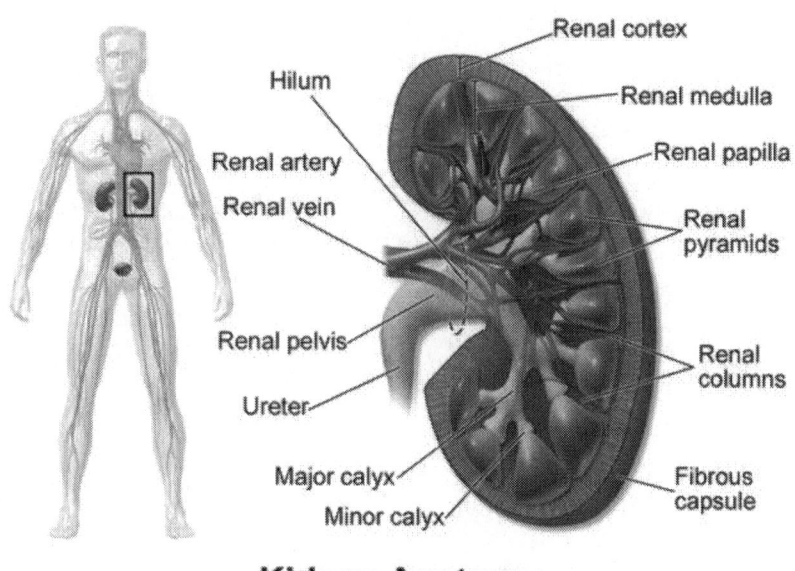

Kidney Anatomy

Basic Anatomy

There are two kidneys in the body. They lie on the right and left side of the abdomen below the liver and stomach respectively. They sit toward the back of the abdomen. An adrenal gland sits directly above each bean shaped kidney. A renal artery enters the kidney and the renal vein and ureter exit the kidney. The functional unit of the kidney is the nephron. The nephron helps filter out excess water and solutes from the blood. Filtered blood then leaves via the renal vein, and waste via the ureter.

Functions

The kidneys play many vital roles in the body including removal of waste products; regulation of blood pressure and electrolytes; acid-base balance; reabsorption of amino acids, glucose, and water; hormone production: calcitriol, erythropoietin; and enzyme production: renin.

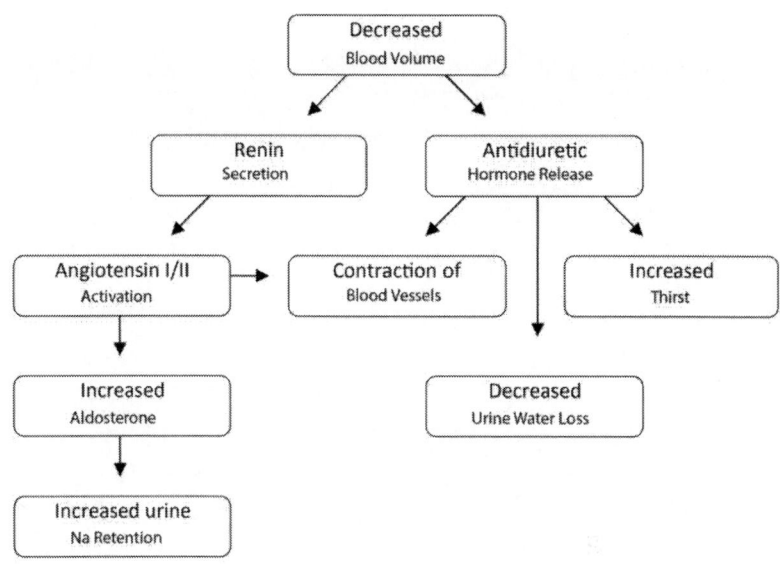

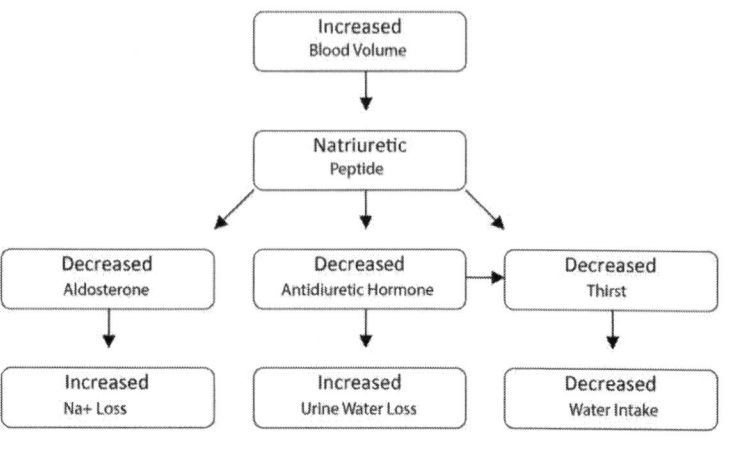

Antidiuretic Hormone (ADH): Stimulated by increased concentration of electrolytes or decreased blood pressure. The hypothalamus has osmoreceptors that monitor osmolarity of the blood. ADH is produced in the hypothalamus and stored in the posterior pituitary gland, it is released from the posterior pituitary into the blood to act on the kidneys. ADH stimulates constriction of blood vessels and water conservation by increasing water reabsorption in the kidneys and decreasing sweat production by sweat glands.

Renin: Created by the kidneys in response to decreased blood flow. Renin stimulates the conversion of angiotensinogen to Angiotensin I, which is then converted to Angiotensin II, via the enzyme angiotensin converting enzyme.

Angiotensin II: Causes blood vessel constriction stimulates aldosterone excretion.

Aldosterone: A hormone made in the kidneys. It works to increase sodium and water reabsorption and increase potassium excretion in urine.

Brain Natriuretic Peptide (BNP): A hormone made in the heart ventricles in response to increase stretching. When stimulated, BNP works to increase sodium and water excretion by the urine. This leads to decreased blood volume and blood pressure.

Atrial Natriuretic Peptide (ANP): A hormone made in the right atrium of the heart in response to increase stretching. Just like BNP, ANP works to increase sodium and water excretion by the urine. This leads to decreased blood volume and blood pressure.

Disorders of Fluid Balance

Hypervolemia

Hypervolemia is an **increase in extracellular fluid** (intravascular and interstitial fluid). In hypervolemia the body compensates with the release of natriuretic peptides- which increase excretion of sodium and water by the kidneys- and inhibition of aldosterone.

Causes

- **Retention of water and sodium**: cirrhosis, nephrotic syndrome, heart failure, excess glucocorticoids

- **Excess fluid administration**: excess IV fluids, excess fluid in total parenteral nutrition

- **Decreased renal function**: acute or chronic renal failure with decreased urine output.

- **Fluid shift from interstitial space to intravascular fluid**: treatment after a burn, hypertonic saline administration, administration of a colloid solution like albumin

Signs & Symptoms

moist skin, edema, ascites, crackles, weight gain, increased blood pressure (decreased BP as heart rate falls), orthopnea, shortness of breath, bounding pulses, wheezes, rhonchi, rales, distended neck veins, tachypnea, tachycardia, gallop rhythm, increased CVP, increased pulmonary artery pressure (PAP), increased pulmonary artery wedge pressure (PAWP), increased mean arterial pressure (MAP) unless pt with heart failure.

Tests

ABGs: identify hypoxemia (decreased PaO_2), and respiratory alkalosis (increased pH and decreased $PaCO_2$)
Chest x-ray: assess for vascular congestion to identify pulmonary congestion.
BNP: increased
BUN: increased in renal failure
Hematocrit: decreased due to dilution
Serum Sodium: decreased in the presence of water retention
Urinary Sodium: possibly elevated if the kidneys are excreting excess sodium.
Urine specific gravity: decreased when kidneys are removing excess fluid

Treatment

Water and sodium restriction: oral, enteral, parenteral

Limit high sodium foods:

Foods High in Sodium

cheese	soy sauce	sauerkraut
canned foods	Olives	snack foods (chips cracker,
boxed meals	Pickles	pretzels).
frozen meal	deli meats	
Ketchup	salad dressings	

Diuretics: IV or oral diuretics, loop diuretics (Furosemide) in severe hypervolemia, or renal failure

Renal replacement therapy (dialysis): in renal failure or very severe volume overload

Monitor

input and output, weight (monitor weights daily, a 2 kg wt gain equals 2 L fluid gain), specific gravity, edema

Hypovolemia

Hypovolemia is a decrease in intravascular fluid/blood volume. With hypovolemia the body will attempt to compensate by increasing stimulation of the central nervous system: increase heart rate, vascular resistance, thirst, ADH, and aldosterone.

Causes

- **Skin:** exercise, fever, burns, or cystic fibrosis.

- **Decreased fluid intake**: coma patient, dementia, limited access to water

- **Renal:** loss of fluid excreted via the kidney can be caused by diabetes mellitus, diabetes insipidus, diuretics, renal disease, and adrenal insufficiency

- **Blood loss**: loss of blood could occur with hemorrhage or surgery

- **Gastrointestinal**: GI loss of fluid due to nausea, vomiting, diarrhea, fistula, nasogastric suction

- **Fluid shift** (from intravascular space into interstitial): peritonitis, small bowel obstruction, pulmonary edema, burns

Signs & Symptoms

sunken eyeballs, increased temp, fatigue, syncope, weight loss, vomiting, increased HR, weakness, constipation, anorexia, thirst, dry tongue, nausea, confusion, oliguria, dizziness, decreased BP, decreased central venous pressure (CVP), decreased pulmonary artery pressure (PAP), decreased cardiac output, decreased mean arterial pressure (MAP), increased systemic vascular resistance

children: decreased tear production, depressed anterior fontanelle, and poor skin turgor.

hypovolemic shock: pale, diaphoretic, rapid thready pulse, oliguria, confusion, decreased blood pressure (BP)

Tests

ABGs: metabolic acidosis secondary to DKA or lower GI loses, and metabolic alkalosis secondary to diuretics, or upper GI losses
BUN: increased, as a result of increased production or decreased excretion (due sodium and water reabsorption)
BUN/creatinine ratio: in hypovolemia BUN will rise more than creatinine. An equal rise in BUN and creatinine is an indicator of renal problems
Hematocrit: increased, due to increased concentration
Serum CO2: increased in metabolic alkalosis, decreased in metabolic acidosis
Serum electrolytes:
    - Potassium: low in GI or renal loss; high in adrenal insufficiency

- Sodium: low due to thirst and increased water intake, high with sweat loss

Serum osmolality: depends on type of fluid lost and amount of compensation

Urine Na: decreased as long as kidney function is normal.

Urine osmolality: increased, increased concentration

Urine specific gravity: increased, more concentrated urine as the body tries to conserve fluid

Treatment

Treatment is based on the type of fluid that is lost. In severe depletion, rapid increase in intravascular fluid is priority.

Treatment with IV Fluids

Crystalloid

- Isotonic Normal Saline: increases intravascular fluid, without increasing intracellular fluid
- Saline/Electrolyte solutions: provides fluid and electrolytes (K+, Ca+, Lactate, acetate)
  - hypotonic fluid is used for maintenance fluids
  - isotonic fluid will replace fluid loss (most fluids lost are isotonic)
- Dextrose solutions: provides free water which is distributed to intracellular fluid and extracellular fluid, replete total body water deficit.

Colloid

- Blood products: increase intravascular fluid only
- Plasma: Increase intravascular fluid

Edema

Edema is an increased volume (swelling) of **interstitial fluid**. Edema can be localized in the case of venous obstruction, or generalized as in heart failure.

Anasarca: severe generalized edema

Causes

- **Increased capillary hydrostatic pressure:** volume expansion, venous obstruction, increased capillary permeability (burns, trauma, allergies, infection), premenstrual syndrome, pregnancy

- **Lymphatic obstruction:** impaired drainage of interstitial fluid

- **Decreased plasma protein concentration** (decreased oncotic pressure): malnutrition, liver disease

- **Increased retention of sodium and water by the kidneys:** renal failure, heart failure, nephrotic syndrome, decreased cardiac output and blood volume cause kidneys to conserve water which leads to an increase in anti-diuretic hormone.

- **Medications:** NSAIDs, steroids, Ca channel blockers

Signs & Symptoms

Fluid retention: in ambulatory patients water is likely to accumulate in the legs or ankle (check for pretibial edema). In a non-ambulatory patient fluid may collect around the sacrum (check for sacral edema).

Generalized edema: will show up around the eyes (periorbital) or scrotal sac secondary to decreased tissue perfusion.

Measure sacral fluid retention: press and hold for several seconds, if pit remains that indicates edema.

Treatment

- Treat the underlying cause: digitalis for congestive heart failure

- Mobilization of edema: bed rest or support hose

- Sodium restriction: avoid medications with sodium

- Renal replacement therapy: renal failure or severe fluid overload.

- Paracentesis: treat severe ascites if it starts to affect the heart and lungs.

- Diuretics:

  - Increased excretion of sodium and water via the kidneys
  - not effective with all edema
  - use with caution with hepatic cirrhosis (decreased electrolytes and circulating volume can lead to hepatic coma, hypokalemia, hepatorenal syndrome

IV Fluids Overview

Treatment for disorders of fluid balance depends on the cause. It is important to understand the different characteristics of IV fluids available. They are useful in different situations.

Crystalloid Solutions

(Download an HD version of this chart at NRSNG.com/IVfluids)

IVF	Content	Tonicity	Osmolality (mOsm/L)	Uses
D5W	-50 g/L glucose -170 kcals/L -no electrolytes	Isotonic	252	-treat hypernatremia, replace water loss -free water (helps renal excretion of solutes) -used to administer medications
D10W	-100 g/L glucose -340 kcals/L -no electrolytes	hypertonic	505	-free water only
½NS	-0.45% saline -77 mMol/L of Na+ and Cl⁻ -no calories	hypotonic	154	-maintenance solution, but doesn't replace other daily electrolytes -free water and NaCl -replace hypotonic fluid loss -can cause IVF overload if infused too rapidly
NS	-0.9% saline -154 mMol/L of Na+ and Cl⁻ -no calories	Isotonic	308	-used for postoperative fluids -increase IVF and replace ECF fluid losses -NaCl in higher concentration then blood levels -no free water -can cause IVF overload -only solution that can be administered with blood products
3%NS	-3.0% saline -513 mMol/L of Na+ and Cl⁻	hypertonic	1026	- administer cautiously, slowly - treatment for symptomatic hyponatremia -cerebral edema
D5- ¼ NS	-0.225% saline -50 g/L glucose -170 kcals/L -38.5 mMol/L of Na+ and Cl⁻	Isotonic	330	-Provides NaCl and free water -treatment for hypernatremia -replace hypotonic fluid loss
D5-½NS	-0.45% saline -50 g/L glucose -170 kcals/L -77 mMol/L of Na+ and Cl⁻	Hypertonic	406	-maintenance solution, but doesn't replace other daily electrolytes -free water and NaCl -replace hypotonic fluid loss -can cause IVF overload if infused too rapidly
D5-NS	-0.9% saline -50 g/L glucose -170 kcals/L -154 mMol/L of Na+ and Cl⁻	Hypertonic	560	-increase IVF and replace ECF fluid losses -used for postoperative fluids -NaCl in higher concentration then blood levels -no free water -can cause IVF overload

(Download an HD version of this chart at NRSNG.com/IVfluids)

Colloid solutions

Colloids consist of blood and blood components: blood, packed red blood cells, fresh frozen plasma, plasma, albumin

Nursing Assessment

Patient History

Medical History:

Look for medical history that might be associated with fluid or electrolyte disturbances

   Medical conditions: Crohn's disease, diabetes mellitus, etc
   Medications: diuretics

Psychological/ Religious/ Cultural History:

Behavioral, emotional, cultural, socioeconomic, or religious disorders that might be associated with fluid or electrolyte disturbances: bulimia, religious fasting, financial constraints that limit purchase of medications etc.

Clinical Assessment

Hemodynamics

Central venous pressure (CVP): Amount of blood returning to right atria. If elevated may indicate fluid overload, pulmonary edema, right sided heart failure. The CVP is measured with a catheter in the right atrium.

Pulmonary artery pressure (PAP): The amount of blood pressure in the pulmonary artery. The PAP is measured via a catheter placed in the pulmonary artery. Increased PAP may indicate increases in fluid volume.

Systemic vascular resistance (SVR): Resistance in peripheral circulation that must be overcome to pump blood to the body.

Cardiac output (CO): The amount of blood pumped out of the heart each minute. heart rate x stroke volume = cardiac output

Mean arterial pressure (MAP): Average pressure in the arteries during one cardiac cycle. It can be calculated using diastolic and systolic blood pressure. MAP = [(2 x diastolic BP)+systolic BP]/3

Heart Rate: A measurement of the number of heart beats in one minute.

Stroke Volume: A measure of blood moved during a contraction of the left ventricle.

Blood Pressure (BP): The pressure exerted on the blood vessels by circulating blood. When blood pressure is decreased it can indicate decrease in fluid volume or possible dysrhythmia from electrolyte abnormalities. Increased blood pressure may indicate increased fluid volume. BP=SVR x CO

Weight

Taking daily weights is an important indicator of fluid status. Weights should be taken at the same time each day using the same scale if possible. Rapid short term weight changes are a sign of fluid status. A weight change of 1 kg is equivalent to a loss or gain of 1 liter of fluid. Total body water gains could be in any of the body compartments.

I/Os

Fluid status can be monitored by measuring daily intake and output of fluid.

Intake: PO fluids (all drinks and foods that are liquid at room temperature), IV Fluids (exact amounts given should be recorded), irrigation (any irrigation that is not pulled back out should be documented), tube feedings (all administered tube feeds and any water flushes).

Output: urine output, profuse sweating, nasogastric tube suction, draining fistula, rapid breathing liquid stool, wound drainage, vomiting

Vital Signs

Body Temp

Elevated temperature leads to increase fluid and electrolyte losses. Fluid volume can also affect temperature: hypovolemia can lead to decreased temperature and vice versa.

Respiratory Rate

Increased respiratory rate leads to increase fluid losses via breathing. Respiratory rate will be elevated in metabolic acidosis. With fluid overload in the lungs crackles or rhonchi may be present.

Heart Rate

Heart rate will increase with decreased fluid volume. In volume overload a bounding pulse is seen. In volume deficit a weak or thready pulse is seen.

Heart rate may be altered with disorders of potassium or magnesium.

Blood Pressure

When blood pressure is decreased it can indicate decrease in fluid volume or possible dysrhythmia from electrolyte abnormalities. Increased blood pressure may indicate increased fluid volume.

Physical Assessment

Integument System

Edema: increases in interstitial volume leads to edema which can be localized or generalized. Bony surfaces like the sacrum or tibia should be used to assess for pitting edema. Edema is rated based on severity 1+ to 4+, with 4+ being most severe.
Skin Moisture: check for flushed and dry skin
Skin Turgor: may indicated changes in interstitial volume, assess by pinching the skin over the forearm, sternum to assess if skin quickly returns to original position.
Tongue: furrowing (rut or groove in the tongue) indicates decrease in fluid volume
Moisture between cheek and tongue: if moisture is decreased it indicates volume deficit

Cardiovascular System

Heart Sounds: The third heart sound (S3) may indicate fluid overload

Veins: the veins in the hands - when the hand is raised hand veins collapse within 3-5 seconds. In fluid volume overload this time may be delayed.

Dysrhythmias: may be related to electrolyte abnormalities: calcium, magnesium, potassium

Neurologic System

Assess reflexes: may be altered with magnesium and calcium abnormalities

Changes in mental status: confusion may be present in hypovolemia, or acid/base imbalances **Trousseau's and Chvostek's sign:** will be positive with decreased calcium or magnesium **Muscular function**: weakness, paralysis can be seen with potassium and calcium deficits

Gastrointestinal System

Anorexia, nausea, vomiting, nasogastric suction are all modes of fluid loss. Increased thirst can be a sign of fluid deficit.

Electrolyte Disorders

Sodium Balance

135-145 mMol/L

Location/Function

Sodium is the main cation in the blood. Small amounts are also found within the cell.

Sodium concentration is important in maintaining the cell **membrane potential**. In excitable cells like neurons and muscle cells, membrane potential is essential for communication and muscle contractions respectively. Sodium also helps maintain fluid balance in the blood. It is the main contributor to osmolality of the blood. Sodium contributes 280 mOsm of the 300 mOsm of the blood. Sodium can move into cells, but is pumped out against electrochemical gradient. Na+ absorption is proportional to intake.

Regulation

Movement from ECF to ICF
If serum sodium increases some sodium will shift into the cell, maintaining the balance of sodium in the blood.

Increase total body sodium
Typical daily intake is usually much higher than our needs.

Excretion
Excretion is regulated by several important hormones: aldosterone, angiotensin II, and natriuretic peptides.

Changes in serum sodium often reflect changes in fluid status. If Na in the blood increases or decreases, the body responds by increasing or decreasing water to maintain sodium concentration. (Remember concentration is affected by both the solute: sodium, and the solvent: water) If you decrease the amount of water you increase concentration. If you increase sodium you increase concentration.   Because the body compensates changes in serum sodium concentration are typically caused by changes in water. This makes sodium a good indicator of hydration.

Hyponatremia

Hyponatremia can be caused by overhydration or body losses of salt water that is replaced with water. The kidneys can compensate be excreting sodium free water. If the body needs to conserve water, however, this compensatory mechanism can't be used. Hyponatremia causes hypoosmolality since sodium plays such a big role in serum osmolality.

When looking at hyponatremia it is important to know if it is in the setting of decreased, increased, or normal ECF volume. In hyponatremia fluid moves out of the blood and into the interstitial spaces.

The brain has a fixed volume due to the skull. Hyponatremia can lead to increased intracranial pressure and cerebral edema. The body adapts over time by decreasing the concentration within the cells of the central nervous system. Neurologic symptoms are higher in acute hyponatremia versus chronic because of this adaptation. If serum sodium levels get below 120 mMol/L neurological symptoms may be seen. Levels below 115 mMol/L can cause seizures or coma.

**It is dangerous to replete sodium too quickly in chronic hyponatremia. It can cause loss of cerebral fluid due to increase in serum osmolality.

Hyponatremia with increased or normal blood volume

Causes

- **Impaired water excretion:** syndrome of inappropriate antidiuretic hormone (SIADH) - increased ADH production, oliguria

- **Fluid shifts:** edema - congestive heart failure, nephrotic syndrome, cirrhosis; hypotonic IV fluids; hyperglycemia leads to a shift of fluid from intracellular to intravascular.

- **Excess fluid intake**: polydispsia (excess thirst)

Sign & Symptoms

muscle weakness, headache, lethargy, apathy, convulsions, confusion, edema, weight gain, elevated BP, muscle cramps, coma, increased mean arterial pressure (MAP), increased, increased central venous pressure (CVP), pulmonary artery pressure (PAP)

Treatment

- Treat underlying cause: SIADH
- Water restriction: 1000 mL/day
- Diuretics: loop diuretics, thiazide diuretics should not be used

In hyponatremia that has persisted for more than 48 hours replete sodium slowly or permanent neurologic damage may occur. No more than 24 mmol/L increase in the first 48 hrs.

Hyponatremia with decreased blood volume

Causes

- **GI loss:** diarrhea, fistula, nasogastric suction, vomiting, laxatives

- **Renal loss:** diuretics, hypoaldosteronism, renal salt wasting

Sign & Symptoms

tremors, personality changes, anxiety, cold skin, irritability, dizziness, postural hypotension, clammy skin, dry mucous membrane seizure, coma, decreased mean arterial pressure (MAP), decreased central venous pressure (CVP), pulmonary artery pressure (PAP), decreased cardiac output, increased systemic vascular resistance

Tests

- **Serum osmolality:** is typically decreased (except is hyperglycemia, azotemia)
- **Serum sodium:** decreased
- **Urine specific gravity:** decreased as kidneys excrete excess fluid
- **Urine sodium:** decreased (except in SIADH and adrenal insufficiency)

Treatment

- Replace sodium, fluid and other electrolytes like potassium and bicarbonate.
- Hypertonic IV solution: 3% NaCl, to correct symptoms, administered with a loop diuretic to prevent fluid overload.

Hypernatremia

Causes

- **Water loss:** conditions that decrease urine concentration (diabetes insipidus), increased insensible loses (respiratory infection, diarrhea)

- **Increased sodium:** hypertonic saline solution, Cushing's syndrome, sodium bicarbonate ($NaHCO_3$), near drowning in salt water, drugs: Kayexalate

- **Inadequate water intake** (issues with thirst or access to water): inadequate fluid administration in coma pt, tube feedings

Signs and Symptoms

During hypernatremia there is decreased tonicity since sodium contributes to osmolality. In response fluid moves out of the cells and into the blood. The cells in the brain adapt by increasing intracellular osmolality. This ensures that the cells won't lose excess water. In chronic hypernatremia this adaptation has occurs, and symptoms are minimal. As with hyponatremia if serum sodium is adjusted too quickly it can damage the adapted neurons. It could case dangerous cerebral edema.

thirst, fatigue, irritability, altered mental status, coma, fever, flushed skin, peripheral edema, postural hypotension, tachycardia and tachypnea, muscle twitching, deep tendon reflexes

- Sodium excess: increased central venous pressure (CVP) and pulmonary artery pressure (PAP)
- Water loss: Decreased central venous pressure (CVP) and pulmonary artery pressure (PAP).

Tests

Dehydration test: hold water for 16-18 hrs, administer ADH, wait 1 hour then check serum and urine osmolality.
Serum osmolality: increased because of increased serum sodium
Serum sodium : increased
Urine specific gravity: increased as kidneys reabsorb water.
Urine osmolality: increased as kidneys reabsorb water.
Urine sodium: decreased with renal water loss

Treatment

- Treat underlying cause: correcting electrolyte imbalance, treat diarrhea or fever.

- Replace water, IV or oral. D5W or hypotonic saline solution, just to replace water deficit.

- Diuretics and oral or IV water replacement

Potassium Balance

3.5 - 5 mEq/L

Location/Function

Potassium is the main cation inside the cell. A small amount of potassium is found in the blood and interstitial fluid.

Potassium is transported into the cell via the sodium-potassium pump. Three sodium ions are pumped out of the cell for every two Potassium ions pumped into the cell. The amount of Potassium outside the cell helps maintain the resting membrane potential. Essentially the outside of the cell is more positive and the inside more negative. The electrical charges separated by the cell membrane give the cells in the body a resting membrane potential. In excitable cells like neurons and muscle cells this membrane potential is essential for communication and muscle contractions respectively.

Regulation

Movement of Potassium from ICF to ECF

Movement between intracellular fluid (ICF) to extracellular fluid (ECF) is affected by insulin, pH, and epinephrine:

Insulin and epinephrine stimulate glucose uptake in to the cells. They also stimulate activity of the Na-K+ pump. The concentration gradient of sodium that is established by the pump allows for the transport of glucose in to the cell.

The pH affects potassium as well. When pH is low, the excess H+ ion in the blood move into the cells. To maintain electric equilibrium potassium moves out of the cell in response. The opposite happens during alkalosis. It is an inverse relationship, as pH goes down potassium goes up and vise versa.

Increased total body Potassium

- Tissue breakdown: since the cell is where most potassium is stored, when cells are broken down that potassium is released into the system.

- Increased Intake: excess potassium rich foods, salt substitutes, transfusions of whole blood or packed red blood cells. Sources of K+ - fruits, vegetables, beans, dairy, meat

- decreased K+ excretion from the kidneys due to K+ sparing diuretics, renal failure, or Addison's disease

Excretion

Potassium is excreted via the kidneys-80%, gastrointestinal tract-15%, and the skin-5%.

The kidneys play a big role in potassium regulation. If intake is high, or tissue catabolism occurs the kidneys will quickly compensate and excrete excess serum potassium via the urine. When plasma potassium concentrations are high the adrenal cortex releases aldosterone which will increase excretion of potassium.

Tip: Aldosterone can also be stimulated by postsurgical stress or volume depletion. In these cases you may also see increase potassium excretion. Lastly increased urine production can also cause increase losses of potassium

Mg def: potassium shifts out of cell, and increased K+ excretion occurs.

Hypokalemia

Causes

- **Inadequate intake**

- **Increased urine production**: aldosterone simulation (volume depletion, surgery, hyperaldosteronism), diuretics, magnesium deficiency

- **Movement of Potassium into the cells**: anabolism, alkalosis, treatment of DKA with insulin, refeeding syndrome, treatment of acidosis-

- **Increased GI losses:** specifically from the stomach, like NGT to suction or pyloric stenosis, vomiting, diarrhea, NG suction, GI surgery

- **Diaphoresis:** excess perspiration

- **Medications:** antibiotics, diuretics, laxatives, insulin, Albuterol, epinephrine

Signs & Symptoms

decreased bowel sounds, vomiting, dysrhythmia, muscle weakness, muscle cramps, fatigue, ileus, nausea, constipation, paralysis, hypoventilation, weak pulse, decreased muscle tone

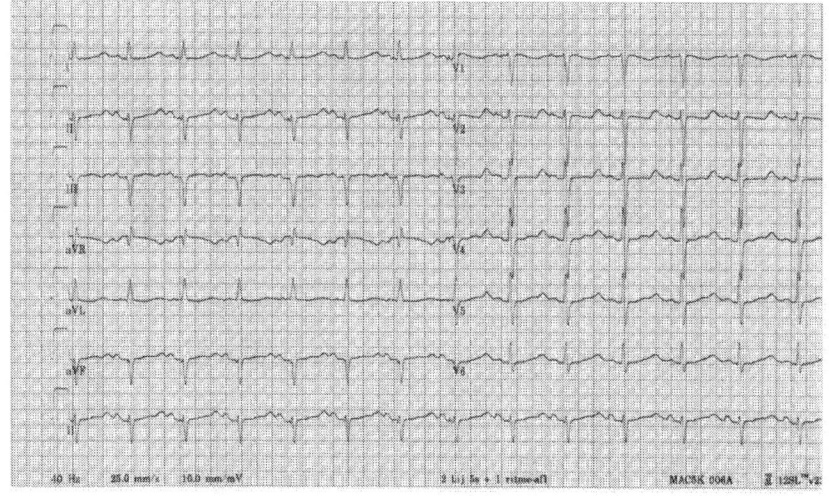

Lab Tests

Serum potassium: decreased
Urine potassium: increased is indicative of renal cause, if decreased cause is not renal.
Transtubular K+ concentration gradient (TTKG): calculated using potassium and osmolaltiy values in the serum and urine to determine cause of increased potassium levels.
ABGs: evaluate acidosis/alkalosis as a possible contributor.
ECG: monitor for ST- segment depression, presence of accentuated U wave, flattened T wave, ventricular dysrhythmias,

Hypokalemia may cause digitalis toxicity even if serum digitalis levels are WNL.

Treatment

- Treat underlying cause

- Increased potassium intake:

Foods High in Potassium

Oranges	Tomatoes	Bananas
Melons	Potatoes	Dried fruit
Nuts	Spinach	Apricots
Avacodos	Chocolate	Dried beans
Peas	Meat	

- Potassium Replacement via oral or IV medication: 40-80 mMol/day IV divided doses. If severe K+ should be replaced via IV: no more than 10-20 mmol/per hour or 30-40mmol/l (unless severe) IV K+ via peripheral line can cause irritation to vessels. Pt on more than 10 mmol/hr should be on continuous cardiac monitor: peaked t wave indicates hyperkalemia. Types: KCl or K phosphate. Usually KCl since vomiting and diuretics cause Cl loss as well. KHCO3 or K citrate if metabolic acidosis is present.

NEVER administer via IV push.

- Potassium sparing diuretics: spironolactone, can help increase serum potassium

- KCl salt substitutes: 1 tsp is equal to 60 mmol KCl

54

- Correct Mg deficiency. If potassium is not improving with significant K+ replacement Mg deficiency might be to blame.

Hyperkalemia

Causes

- **Intake:** excess IV potassium administration

- **Movement of potassium out of cells**
  -insulin deficiency (esp with patients that also have chronic renal insufficiency)
  -acidosis (metabolic and respiratory)
  -tissue breakdown due to fever, sepsis, trauma, surgery
  -hypertonicity (uncontrolled DM)

- **Excretion:**
  -renal failure
  -potassium sparing diuretics, ACE inhibitors, NSAIDs
  -adrenal insufficiency
  -Addison's disease

- **Medications:** potassium sparing diuretics, ACE inhibitors, beta blockers, chemotherapy medications, heparin, digoxin, NSAIDs

In **DKA** potassium in the blood can be elevated despite increased loss of potassium in the urine. During the lack of insulin, acidosis, and increased catabolism potassium moves out of the cells into the blood.

Signs & Symptoms

respiratory distress, diarrhea, irritability, anxiety, muscle weakness, paresthesia, abdominal cramping, anuria, ECG changes, hyperreflexia

Tests

ABGs: identify acidosis as possible cause of hyperkalemia
Diagnostic ECG: monitor for prolonged PR interval, ST depression, thin T wave, widened QRS, and loss of P wave.
Serum Cortisol: identify Addison's disease
Serum Potassium: elevated
Transtubular K+ concentration gradient (TTKG): calculated using potassium and osmolaltiy values in the serum and urine to determine cause of increased potassium levels.

Treatment

Medications:
  -Kayexalate: Kayexalate is a resin that binds to
    potassium in the colon so that it is excreted.
  -Fludrocortisone: increases urinary excretion of
  potassium
  -Calcium gluconate IV can help counteract the
   cardiac and neurologic effects of hyperkalemia.
  -IV glucose and insulin: this will help shift
    potassium from the blood and into the cells.
    The effect lasts about 6 hours

-Sodium bicarbonate: this will help shift
   potassium into the cells. The effect lasts 1-2
   hours
-Beta2 agonists: this will help shift potassium into
the cell. (Albuterol)

Limit potassium intake: following a low potassium
diet or choosing an enteral product with less
potassium

Discontinue medications that might be contributing
to hyperkalemia: NSAIDs, ACE inhibitors,
potassium-sparing diuretics

Dialysis: removes potassium from the body.

Calcium

Location/Function

Calcium is stored in the bones and teeth. Calcium
Phosphorus salts help give bones their strength.
Sodium is found in the ECF but less than 1% of
total body Calcium is there. Calcium plays a very
important role in muscle contraction, and has an
inhibitory affect on neurons.

Regulation

There are several mechanisms that help maintain
the amount of calcium in the blood. When levels of
calcium are low parathyroid hormone is released
from the parathyroid gland. PTH acts to breakdown
bone so that the stored calcium can replete calcium

in the ECF. PTH also activates Vitamin D which increase calcium absorption from the intestines. Active Vitamin D also stimulates the kidneys to conserve calcium and excrete phosphorus. When calcium levels are too high the thyroid gland releases calcitonin. Calcitonin stops bone breakdown. Both dietary intake and bone breakdown can lead to increase in calcium levels Calcium is lost in gastrointestinal secretions, urinary excretion, bone deposition, and sweat (in small amounts). Typically we only absorb 20-30% of dietary calcium.

Hypocalcemia

Causes

- **Increased calcium loss:** diuretics

- **Decreased intake:** decreased absorption (diarrhea, gastric surgery), reduced intake, vitamin D deficiency,

- **Altered regulation**
  - hypoparathyroidism.
  - hyperphosphatemia (rhabdomyolysis, renal failure, tumor lysis syndrome) elevated phosphorus can lead to low calcium. Calcium and phosphorus have a reciprocal relationship, as one goes up the other goes down.
  -hypomagnesemia
  -Thyroidectomy (calcium moves from blood back into bone)

- Acute pancreatitis, chronic alcoholism, bone cancer, alkalosis

Since some Calcium in the blood is bound to protein (albumin), when albumin is low total calcium may be low. This is not a problem and doesn't need treatment as long as ionized Calcium is within normal limits.

Signs and Symptoms

arrhythmias, numbness, tingling fingers, hyperactive reflexes, muscle cramps, tetany, convulsions, tetany, stridor and spasms, lethargy, anxiety, depression, psychosis, decreased heart contractility and heart failure, positive chvostek's sign and trousseau's sign

ECG changes: prolonged QT, elongation of ST segment--> ventricle tachycardia.

Tests

Ionized serum Ca: decreased - most useful measure to detect calcium deficiency
Magnesium: low Mg may cause low Ca
Parathyroid hormone: Decreased levels indicate hypoparathyroidism which is related to low calcium
Phosphorus: elevated Phos may cause low Ca
Total serum Ca: total Calcium in the blood may be declined due to decreased protein that calcium is bound to. Look at albumin levels and pH when assessing for deficiency

Treatment

Treat the underlying cause:

- Replete calcium: This can be done orally or via IV. With symptoms present usually IV calcium gluconate is best option.
- Replete magnesium: If Mg is the cause of deficiency, replace.
- Vitamin D: Vitamin D increases absorption of Calcium if repleting calcium orally.
- Phosphate binder: This can help reduce elevated phosphorus levels in patients with renal failure.
- Increased intake: replete via oral intake: 1000-1500 mg/ day
- Oral supplements: calcium carbonate

Foods High in Calcium

Milk	Collard greens	Yogurt
Cheese	Oats	Tofu
Broccoli	Rhubarb	Salmon
Ice cream	Soy flour	
Mustard	Spinach	

Hypercalcemia

Causes

- **Increased intake:** Excess IV calcium

- **Decreased excretion:** renal failure, thiazide diuretics

- **Bone breakdown:** prolonged immobility, fractures, malignant diseases, Paget's disease, hyperparathyroidism, hyperthyroidism, hypophosphatemia

- **Increase absorption:** Vitamin D or Vitamin A overdose

- **Medications:** diuretics, ace inhibitors

Signs & Symptoms

weakness, lethargy, nausea, vomiting, anorexia, polyuria (from nephrogenic diabetes insipidus), bone pain, fractures, itching, flank pain (renal calculi), confusion, depression, stupor, coma, personality changes, paresthesia, ECG findings: shortening of ST segment and QT interval, prolonged PR interval. more severe: ventricular dysrhythmia. Risk for digitalis toxicity

Lab Tests

Imaging: assess bone density, identify kidney stones
Ionized Calcium: elevated
Parathyroid hormone: increased in hyperparathyroidism
Serum Calcium: elevated, assess serum albumin level: for every 1g/dL drop in albumin there is a drop in calcium of 0.8- 1 mg/dL decrease in serum calcium

Treatment

Treat underlying cause: partial parathyroidectomy for hyperparathyroidism, chemotherapy for malignant disease, or discontinue ca supplements, vitamin A, vitamin D, thiazide diuretics in renal patients

IV NS solution: Administer rapidly to increased Ca excretion via urine. Administer diuretics at the same time to prevent volume overload and to increase calcium excretion.

Low calcium diet: limit calcium intake.

Medications:
- Bisphosphates: Pamidronate or etidronate: These medications inhibit bone resorption. This medication is most often used for malignant disease
- Plicamycin: cytotoxic antibiotics that decreases bone resorption. Used with neoplastic disorders.
- Calcitonin: Reduces bone resorption and increase bone deposition of Ca and phos. increase urinary ca and phosphorus excretion.
- Gallium nitrate: inhibit bone resorption - used in malignant disease.
- Cortisone: Steroids compete with Vitamin D for absorption in the small intestines. This decreases calcium absorption as well.

Hemodialysis: with low calcium dialysate in renal failure patients

Phosphorus

2.5-4.5 mg/dL   0.81 – 1.45 mMol/L

Location/Function

Phosphorus is the main anion in inside the cell. The majority of Phosphorus is stored with Calcium in bones and teeth - 85%. The inside of the cell contains 14% of phosphorus, and the blood has about 1%. Most phosphorus in the body is in the form of phosphate.

Functions
- Essential for nerve and muscle function
- Involved in acid/base balance
- Formation of red blood cells
- Component of ATP (important form of stored energy in the body)
- Carbohydrate, protein, fat metabolism
- A part of structure of bones and teeth

Regulation

Decrease phosphorus: insulin, glucose, carbohydrate (phosphorus shifts into the cell due to increased needs for of phosphorus during metabolism), alkalosis, specifically respiratory alkalosis due to intracellular shift of phosphorus

Increase phosphorus: respiratory acidosis can cause shift of phosphorus out of cell, increased intake, intestinal absorption increased, bone reabsorption, impaired renal excretion.

PTH causes increased GI absorption, increased movement of phosphorus out of bone. PTH also increases renal excretion.

Close relationship between calcium and phosphorus

Hypophosphatemia

Causes

- **Inadequate intake:** TPN with inadequate phosphorus

- **Intracellular fluid shifts:** insulin, carbohydrate load, respiratory alkalosis, androgen therapy, refeeding syndrome, malnutrition

- **Tissue repair:** phosphorus is needed to help with energy supply during tissue repair

- **Increased Excretion:** decreased magnesium, decreased potassium, hyperparathyroidism, thiazide diuretics, ATN, Fanconi's syndrome

- **Decreased absorption or intestinal loss:** phosphorus binding antacids (aluminum, calcium, magnesium), vomiting, nasogastric suction, diarrhea, malabsorption, vitamin D deficiency

- **Combination:** Alcohol, alcohol withdrawal, DKA treatment, severe burns.

- **Medications:** phosphate binders, antacids, diuretics, laxative abuse

Signs & Symptoms

Acute : coma, decreased grip strength, lack of coordination, seizures, chest pain secondary to poor oxygenation, muscle pain, increased risk of infection, confusion, numbness tingling of fingers and circumoral region, difficulty weaning from the vent, decreased strength: difficulty speaking, respiratory muscle weakness (the weakenss in th respiratory muscles can lead to hypoxemia and hyperventilation which may lead to respiratory alkalosis which aggravates the hypophosphatemia), bleeding due to platelet dysfunction, rhabdomyolysis and hemolysis in severe cases.

Chronic: joint pain, weakness, pseudo fractures, lethargy, memory loss, cyanosis, joint stiffness, osteomalacia

Lab Tests

Serum Phosphorus: decreased (moderate: 1-2.5 mg/dL, severe: < 1mg/dL)
PTH: identify hyperparathyroidism
Serum Magnesium: may be decreased due to increased excretion during hypophosphatemia
Alkaline Phosphatase: increased during building of bones (osteoblast activity)
Imaging: identify changes in bone density, shape: osteomalacia, rickets

Treatment

- Treat underlying cause: avoid phosphate binders (aluminum, magensium, calcium antacids)

- Increase Phosphorus intake: consume high Phos foods (meat organ meats especially, fish, poultry, milk, dairy, whole grains, seeds, nuts, eggs, dried beans/peas), take and oral supplement: NeutraPhos, IV phosphorus if severe: NaPhos or KPhos.

Foods High in Phosphorus

organ meats	whole grains	dried beans
fish	Seeds	dried peas
poultry	nuts	
dairy	eggs	

Hyperphosphatemia

Causes

- **Decreased excretion:** hypoparathyroidism, acute or chronic renal failure, volume depletion.

- **Increased intake:** vitamin D excess with increased GI absorption, fertilizer poisoning, excess administration of phosphorus supplements, excess use of Phosphorus containing laxatives or enemas

- **Extracellular shifts:** respiratory acidosis and metabolic acidosis, diabetic ketoacidosis, infection

- **Movement of phosphorus out of cells:** Neoplastic disease (leukemia, lymphoma), increased tissue catabolism (trauma, crush injury), tumor lysis syndrome, chemotherapy, rhabdomyolysis (breakdown of striated muscle)

Signs & Symptoms

tetany, muscle weakness, nausea, vomiting, anorexia, tachycardia, hyperreflexia

Most symptoms associated with hyperphosphatemia are actually associated with the accompanying hypocalcemia that often occurs. Other symptoms may occur in metastatic disease due to soft tissue calcification: corneal haziness, conjunctivitis, oliguria, irregular HR, and papular eruptions.

Tests

Blood urea nitrogen (BUN): assess renal status
Creatinine: assess renal status
Imaging: assess bone density: osteodystrophy
Parathyroid hormone: decreased - identify hyperparathyroidism
Serum calcium: help identify primary cause

Serum phosphorus: increased

Treatment

Treat underlying cause: correct volume depletion, treat secondary hyperparathyroidism in chronic renal failure: in chronic renal failure excess PTH can lead to elevated phosphorus and bone disease. Vitamin D can help reduce PTH levels.

Limit Phosphorus intake: avoid high phosphorus foods.

Phosphate binders: (Renvela) Phosphate binders bind to Phosphorus in the GI tract to decrease absorption.

Antacids to bind phosphorus (Aluminum, Calcium, or Magnesium antacids): These medications will bind to phosphorus and decrease absorption. In renal failure Calcium is preferred to Magnesium or Aluminum.

Dialysis: Dialysis may be necessary in severe acute hyperphosphatemia, with symptomatic hypocalcemia.

Magnesium

1.5-2.5 mEq/L

Location/Function

The majority of magnesium is stored in the bone, 50-60%. Only 1% of magnesium is in the blood, and the remainder is inside the cell.

Magnesium activates enzymes that breakdown carbohydrate and protein, triggers the Na/K pump, and plays a role is neuron communication and heart function. Most of Magnesium in the blood is ionized, but there is a portion bound to protein.

Regulation

Absorption of magnesium is controlled by vitamin D. Excretion is regulated by the kidneys. Excretion is affected by 3 things: excretion of sodium and calcium, blood volume, and parathyroid hormone.

$\uparrow$ PTH $\rightarrow \downarrow$ Mg Excretion
$\downarrow$ Sodium and Calcium excretion $\rightarrow \downarrow$ Mg Excretion
$\downarrow$ blood volume $\rightarrow \downarrow$ Mg Excretion

Hypomagnesemia

Causes

- **Decreased intake:** decreased GI absorption-malabsorption

- **Shift of magnesium into cell**

- **Increased magnesium excretion:** diuretics

- **Excess GI loss** (vomiting, diarrhea, nasogastric suction, fistula)

- alcoholism, cirrhosis, hyperthyroidism, hypothyroidism, pancreatitis, preeclampsia, hemodialysis, hypercalcemia, hypothermia, burns, sepsis, wound debridement

Signs & Symptoms

paresthesia, insomnia, loss of appetite, mood changes, confusion, fatigue, weakness, hallucinations

Tests

ECG: may see changes related to magnesium, potassium or calcium deficiencies.
Serum Albumin: if albumin is decreased it may cause decreased magnesium level
Serum Calcium: decreased - due to decreased action of PTH caused by
Serum Ionized Mg: decreased - tends to reflect intracellular magnesium
Serum Magnesium: decreased (can be normal despite low intracellular magnesium)
Serum Potassium: decreased - hypokalemia may be resistant to replacement if the cause is a problem with the sodium-potassium pump - magnesium may need to be repleted first
hypomagnesemia
Urine Mg: identify renal cause

Treatment

- oral Mag-Ox in mild or chronic hypomagnesemia

- IV or IM mgSo4 in sever hypomagnesaemia
- add to TPN if pt receiving IV nutrition
- increased dietary intake:

Foods High in Magnesium

Meat	seeds	Oranges
seafood	chocolate	dark green leafy vegetables
Legumes	coconuts	
nuts	bananas	

Hypermagnesemia

Causes

- **Increased intake:** antacids laxatives that contain magnesium, enemas, laxatives, excess admin of IV MgSo4, excess magnesium in TPN

- **Decreased excretion:** renal failure, adrenocortical insufficiency (Addison's disease, hypothermia)

- Untreated DKA, cortical insufficiency, hemodialysis using magnesium rich dialysate

Signs & Symptoms

sensation of heat, decreased deep tissue reflexes, soft tissue calcification, hypotension, weakness, nausea, vomiting, decreased arterial pressure, bradycardia, lost knee jerk reflex (patellar reflex), diaphoresis, coma, flushing, altered mental function, drowsiness, paralysis, paralysis of respiratory muscles may occur when Mg > 10 mEq/L

Tests
ECG: AV block, prolonged QT interval

Serum Magnesium: increased

Treatment

Treat underlying cause: if magnesium is high due to medication, d/c the medication (antacids or laxatives that have magnesium: Maalox, Mylanta, Mag Citrate, Milk of Magnesia, Mag-Sulfate)

Diuretics and 0.45% normal saline: will help increase magnesium excretion, as long as patient has adequate renal function.

IV Ca gluconate: counteract neuromuscular effects of Mg if Hypermagnesemia is severe.

Dialysis with a low magnesium dialysate (pt with severe renal impairment)

Acid Base Balance

To understand acid/base balance in the body first an overview of acids and bases.

Acid: An acid is a substance that donates a hydrogen ion when dissolved in water.

Base: A base binds with hydrogen ions in water.

pH is inversely related to the number of free hydrogen ions in the blood. The more hydrogen ions, the lower the pH and the more acidic a solution. A neutral pH is 7.4 which is the pH of water.

Normal pH in the body ranges from 7.35 - 7.45.

In the body there are several big contributors to the pH of the blood. The following equation shows the relationship between those contributors. H2CO3 is also known as carbonic acid.

$$CO_2 + H_2O <---> H_2CO_3^- <---> H^+ + HCO_3^-$$

Acid Base Balance

If the pH in the blood decreases this is called acidosis; an increase in pH is called alkalosis. Changes in pH can do damage to body cells and tissues. For protection the body has several mechanisms to immediately respond to and correct changes in pH. This helps the body compensate quickly to changes.

pH Regulation

Buffers

There are buffers in all different fluids in the body. If excess acid or base is present, buffers are chemicals that can bind to the acid or base to neutralize their effect on pH. Buffers work as long as the amount of excess acid or base does not exceed that of the buffer binding capacity. There are several important buffers in the body:

Bicarbonate: Bicarbonate has the greatest role in the body as a buffer. It is found in large quantity throughout the body. HCO_3 is produced by the kidneys and aids in excretion of excess hydrogen in the blood.

Proteins: Proteins are present in cells and in the blood. Hemoglobin functions as a buffer.

Ammonium (NH_4^+): Ammonia (NH_3) is created by the kidneys. It can pick up a hydrogen ion to form ammonium. Ammonium is then excreted by the kidneys.

Phosphate: Phosphate assists with excretion of excess hydrogen ions via the kidneys.

Respiratory System

When hydrogen ion concentration is abnormal it is detected by the brain. One of the first mechanisms of action is on the respiratory system. During acidosis alveolar ventilation increases, and decreases with alkalosis. This response can occur within minutes of detection. With increase ventilation the body can help remove CO_2, or conserve CO_2 in the case of alkalosis. If the lungs are healthy they are 50-70% effective at correcting pH imbalances.

Renal System

The kidneys can help regulate acid base balance by controlling the amount of HCO_3- in the blood. When CO_2 levels are elevated the kidneys respond by excreting hydrogen ions. When hydrogen is excreted the kidneys produce $HCO_3$to maintain the balance. During alkalosis the kidneys retain hydrogen ions and excrete HCO_3. The response by the kidneys can take hours to days, but is very effective. The kidneys can excrete large amounts of HCO_3 or $H+$ from the blood and help return pH to a safe range.

Tests

Arterial Blood Gases (ABGs): pH, $PaCO_2$, total CO_2, PaO_2, base excess, saturation
Base Excess: measure of the amount of hydrogen ion required to bring the pH back to 7.35 if pCO_2 were normal
PaCO2: Partial pressure of CO_2 in arteries. CO_2 is the major respiratory component of acid base

balance. The rate and depth of ventilation affect amount of CO_2 in the blood

PaO2: Oxygen does not directly affect acid/base balance, but respiratory function does. Levels of PaO2 can indicate hypoxemia which can lead to metabolic acidosis (due to lactic acid). Hypoxemia can also lead to hyperventilation which can cause respiratory alkalosis

pH: serum hydrogen ion concentration. pH: 7.4 is normal, elevated indicates alkalosis, lower indicates acidosis. Due to compensation mechanisms, the pH may be normal even when there may be a disturbance to acid/bas balance

Saturation: measurement of hemoglobin saturation by oxygen

Total CO2 (HCO3): bicarbonate is the major metabolic component of acid base balance. The kidneys regulate bicarbonate levels in the blood

Acid Base Disorders

Acute Metabolic Acidosis

Metabolic acidosis is a decrease in serum bicarbonate.

$$pH < 7.4 \qquad HCO3^- < 24 \ mEq/L$$

The body compensates very quickly via the respiratory system. A decreased pH stimulates respirations which leads to a decreased paCO2. The buffer system and kidneys will also try to compensate, but acids may build up more quickly than the body can compensate for.

Causes

- **Renal disease:** acute renal failure, renal tubular acidosis

- **Loss of base (alkali):** draining wounds (pancreatic fistula), diarrhea, ureterostomy, cholestyramine, biliary and pancreatic drainage, ileostomy

- **Ketoacidosis:** diabetes mellitus, alcoholism, starvation

- **Lactic acidosis:** Respiratory or circulatory failure, drugs, toxins, septic shock, leukemia, tumors, pancreatitis, uncontrolled DM.

- **Drug toxicity:** salicylates, ammonium chloride, methamphetamine, methanol, ethylene, glycol, poisoning, ecstasy, cocaine

Signs & Symptoms

confusion, fatigue, stupor, headache, nausea, vomiting, diarrhea, coma, decreased blood pressure, tachypnea, alveolar hyperventilation (Kussmaul's respirations), cold and clammy skin, presence of dysrhythmias, shock

Tests

ABGs: decreased pH, monitor PaCO2 to determine amount of respiratory compensation
ECG: identify problems associated with hyperkalemia: depressed ST segment, decreased P wave, peaked T wave, widened QRS complex, decreased R wave
Serum electrolytes: acidosis can cause elevated potassium and chloride
Total CO2 (HCO3): decreased

Treatment

Treat underlying conditions

- Lactic acidosis: correct the underlying cause, NaHCO3 may worsen acidosis if tissue hypoxia is present. If used should be given in small amounts and monitored closely.
- Diarrhea: correct multiple electrolyte imbalances
- Acute renal failure: hemodialysis or peritoneal dialysis to restore plasma bicarbonate
- Renal tubular acidosis: may require treatment with bicarbonate
- DKA: treat with insulin fluids, NaHCO3 (if pH is very low)
- Alcohol: treat with glucose and saline, monitor phosphorus for refeeding syndrome: severe drop in phosphorus can occur 12-24 hours after treatment
- Drug toxicity: depending on the drug hemodialysis may be necessary

Sodium bicarbonate: used when pH is below 7.1, administered via IV
-careful to prevent hypernatremia, metabolic alkalosis, hypokalemia, pulmonary edema, check ABGs and HCO3at least 30 minutes after infusion.

Potassium: hyperkalemia is present usually, but deficit can occur. Potassium needs to be corrected before administering NaHCO3 - when acidosis is corrected potassium shifts into cells.

Mechanical ventilation: respiratory rate on the vent should not be set lower than spontaneous respiratory rate. Large enough tidal volume to allow compensatory hyperventilation until the cause is resolved.

Chronic Metabolic Acidosis

Causes: typically related to chronic renal failure

Signs & Symptoms: generally asymptomatic but sometimes lethargy, fatigue, anorexia

Tests
ABGs: decreased pH, decreased $PaCO_2$
Serum electrolytes: correction of acidosis can lead to hypocalcemia and hypokalemia
Total CO2 (HCO3): decreased

Treatment: dialysis, alkalizing agent (NaHCO3) to maintain bicarbonate (use cautiously to avoid hypocalcemia), limit protein intake

Acute Metabolic Alkalosis

Elevated serum bicarbonate

$$pH > 7.4 \qquad HCO3^- \ (Total\ CO2) > 24\ mEq/L$$

Loss of hydrogen ions or excess alkali intake. Alkalosis is usually caused by potassium depletion of chloride depletion

Causes

- **Volume depletion:** vomiting, bulimia, gastric drainage, thiazide diuretics

- **Aldosteronism:** primary (adenoma) or secondary (severe hypertension, renal cell cancer or mineral-corticoid excess)

- **Post hypercapneic alkalosis**: chronic CO2 retention is rapidly corrected, the HCO3 is still present and can lead to alkalosis

- **Excess alkali intake:** iatrogenic, over correction of metabolic acidosis - seen with CPR, excess ingestion of NaHCO3 (Alka-Seltzer, Tums, Rolaids) especially in renal insufficiency.

- laxative abuse or clay ingestion

Signs & Symptoms

muscular weakness, neuromuscular instability, hyporeflexia, polyuria, polydypsia (secondary to hypokalemia), signs of volume depletion: postural hypotension, decreased jugular venous pressure, poor skin turgor, ECG changes can occur: atrial ventricular dysrhythmias secondary to hypokalemia, changes to T and U waves.

Severe: tetany, confusion, apathy, stupor

Tests

ABGs: increased pH, increased PaCO2 (unless lung disease is present)
ECG: changes associated with hypokalemia
Serum electrolytes: decreased potassium and chloride
HCO3(Total CO2): increased
Urine electrolytes: might be helpful in identifying cause of metabolic alkalosis

Treatment

Treat based on underlying cause, however mild to moderate metabolic alkalosis often does not need treatment

Saline infusion: isotonic infusion may correct volume chloride deficit in patients with alkalosis from gastric losses, diuretics, post hypercapnia
Difficult to correct to hypovolemia and chloride deficit are not corrected.

Chronic metabolic alkalosis

Causes: mineral-corticoids - cause decrease excretion of HCO3 , loss of H+ through the gastrointestinal tract, diuretics

Signs & Symptoms: may be asymptomatic, if severe possibly weakness, decreased GI motility, neuromuscular instability, premature ventricular contractions with hypokalemia and alkalosis.

Lab Tests
ABGs: increased pH, increased PaCO2
Serum electrolytes: decreased potassium, magnesium, and chloride
HCO3(Total CO2): increased

Treatment: replete potassium (IV supplementation, oral supplementation, increased intake), IV fluids (isotonic saline), potassium sparing diuretics, treatment for hyperadrenocorticism

Lungs will compensate and PaCO2 will be elevated.

Respiratory Acidosis

A decrease in carbon dioxide due to alveolar hypoventilation

pH < 7.4   PaCO2 > 40 mm Hg

Causes

Respiratory disease: pneumonia, adult respiratory distress syndrome, acute exacerbation of underlying lung disease (COPD or asthma), chest wall trauma (flail chest, pneumothorax), hemothorax, smoke inhalation, massive pulmonary embolus, severe pulmonary edema

Overdose of drugs: oversedation, anesthesia, respiratory center depression, toxins

CNS trauma/lesions: can lead to depression of respiratory center - cerebral infarct

Asphyxiation: mechanical obstruction, anaphylaxis, aspiration

Impaired respiratory muscles: hypokalemia, Guillain-Barre syndrome, myasthenia gravis crisis

Electrolyte abnormality: severe hypercalcemia, hypokalemia, hypophosphatemia,

Iatrogenic: inappropriate mechanical ventilation

Signs and Symptoms

psychosis with hallucinations, restlessness, confusion, irritability, diaphoresis, lethargy, delusions, and delirium, anxiety, increased heart rate and respiratory rate, cyanosis, severe hypercapnia might cause cerebral vasodilation, increased intracranial pressure, papilledema, dilated facial blood vessels, CNS depression

Tests

ABGs: decreased pH, increased PaCO2
Chest x-ray: identify respiratory disease
Serum electrolytes: typically stable
HCO3 (Total CO2): initially normal

Treatment

Treat underlying cause

Restore normal PH: With PaO2 is greater than 50-60 mm Hg will lead to cyanosis and lethargy. Patient may need intubation and mechanical ventilation. NaHCO3 is usually avoided secondary to risk of alkalosis once respiratory disturbance has been corrected. Small amount of NaHCO3 may be given in severe cases, small doses over 10-15 minutes, and close monitoring.

Chronic respiratory acidosis

Causes: COPD (emphysema, bronchitis), pulmonary toxins, morbid obesity

Signs & Symptoms: body will compensate and a patient may be asymptomatic, possible symptoms: lethargy, weakness, insomnia, headache, agitation, flapping tremor, hypercapnia, coma

Tests
ABGs: slightly decreased pH, increased PaCO2
Chest x-ray: identify respiratory disease

HCO3 (Total CO2): increased due to compensation, if not elevated may indicated multiple causes of acidosis

Treatment: IV fluids, medications (bronchodilators and antibiotics), oxygen therapy, chest physiotherapy

Respiratory Alkalosis

$pH > 7.4$ $PaCO2 < 40$ mm Hg

Causes

- Anxiety may lead to hyperventilation

- Hypoxemia: Pulmonary disorders: asthma, pneumonia, pulmonary edema, pulmonary thromboembolism, heart failure, inhalation of irritants

- Metabolic states: fever, sepsis, septicemia, hepatic disease, hormones (progesterone)

- Salicylate intoxication

- Excessive mechanical ventilation

- Central nervous system trauma: tumors, stroke, trauma can lead to respiratory damage

Signs and Symptoms

dizziness, vertigo, anxiety, euphoria, paresthesia, palpitations, circumoral numbness, chest pain, nausea, vomiting, increased respiratory rate

severe: syncope, tetany, seizures

Tests

ABGs: increased pH, decreased $PaCO_2$
ECG: alkalosis can cause cardiac dysrhythmia
Serum electrolytes: hyperkalemia early on, hypophosphatemia
HCO3 (Total CO2): normal, if elevated may indicated multiple causes of acidosis

Treatment

- Treat underlying cause

- Reassurance: breathing into a paper bag can help increase PCO_2 inhalation, oxygen mask with attached CO_2 reservoir

- Oxygen: if hypoxemia is the cause

- Adjust mechanical ventilation: adjusted based on results of ABGs.

- Pharmacotherapy: sedatives and tranquilizers can help with anxiety

Chronic respiratory alkalosis

Causes: encephalitis, fibrosis, chronic hypoxemia, pregnancy, chronic hepatic insufficiency, tumor, hormone replacement therapy

Signs & Symptoms: kidneys will start to compensate and usually a patient is asymptomatic, but may increased rate and depth of respirations

Tests
ABGs: slightly increased pH, decreased PaCO2
Serum electrolytes: hypophosphatemia
HCO3 (Total CO2): decreased due to compensation

Treatment: treat underlying cause, oxygen therapy

Acid Base Summary

If PaCO2 is the cause: ↑ PaCO2 will cause in ↓ pH and ↓ PaCO2 will cause ↑ pH - inverse relationship

If HCO3is the cause: ↑ HCO3 will cause in ↑ pH and ↓ HCO3will cause ↓ pH - direct relationship

In Simple acidosis an elevated PaCO2 indicates a respiratory cause, and decreased HCO3indicates metabolic cause. CO2 is regulated by the lungs, and HCO3 is regulated by the kidneys.

Compensation: During Respiratory acidosis the kidneys will start to compensate. The kidneys will conserve HCO3 to raise the pH back within a normal range.

Instructions for Chart Below

1. **Alkalosis/Acidosis:** note the pH: low pH indicates acidosis, high pH indicates alkalosis

2. **Metabolic/Respiratory:** look at PaCO2 and HCO3.   An inverse relationship between pH and PaCO2 indicates a respiratory cause of pH disturbance. A direct relationship between pH and HCO3 indicates a metabolic cause.

3. **Compensation:** If the cause is respiratory there will be a metabolic compensation. The compensation will be a response that will change the pH in the opposite way. In acidosis a decreased PaCO2 would cause acidosis, indicating respiratory cause. HCO3would then be conserved and so we see an increase which increases the pH.

	pH	PaCO2	HCO3-
Simple Metabolic Acidosis	↓	--	↓
Compensated Metabolic Acidosis	↓	↓	↓
Simple Respiratory Acidosis	↓	↑	--
Compensated Respiratory Acidosis	↓	↑	↑

Mixed Acidosis	↓	↑	↓
Simple Metabolic Alkalosis	↑	--	↑
Compensated Metabolic Alkalosis	↑	↑	↑
Simple Respiratory Alkalosis	↑	↓	--
Compensated Respiratory Alkalosis	↑	↓	↓
Mixed Alkalosis	↑	--	↑

Sample:

pH: 7.27
PaCO2: 22 mmHg
HCO3-: 9 mEq/L

Steps:

1. In this case the pH is below the normal 7.4. Since the pH is low we are looking at acidosis.

2. The PaCO2 of 22 mmHg is below the normal 40 mmHg. The HCO3 of 9 mEq/L is below normal 24 mEq/L. Decreased PaCO2 increases pH, while decreased HCO3 decreases pH. The cause of the acidosis is therefore metabolic.

3. The PaCO2 being decreased is an indicator that the lungs are attempting to bring the pH back to normal by exhaling extra CO2.

Case Study 1

History:

NW is a 46 year old male with a history of hypertension, chronic alcoholism, anxiety/depression, and dyslipidemia. Recently he has had nausea, vomiting, and right upper quadrant abdominal pain for 3 months. Patient reports 25 lb wt loss over the past 3 months. Typical alcohol consumption prior to recent symptoms was 15 beers a day, more recently he has been drinking vodka with sweet and sour. The day of admit he noticed he was jaundiced. He saw a gastroenterologist a couple months ago who recommended an EGD. The EGD has not yet been completed.

Labs:

Labs		4/5	4/5	4/6
Na	135-145 mMol/L	124		130
K	3.5 - 5 mEq/L	6.3	3.9	4
Cl	98-107 mEq/L	87		91
CO2	21-32 mEq/L	26		33

BUN	7-18 mg/dL	11		6
Creat	0.6-1.3 mg/dL	0.7		1
Ca	8.4-10.2 mg/dL	6.7		8
Glucose	70-99 mg/dL	166		157
Albumin	3.5-6 g/dL	1.9		2.2
AST	15-37 U/L	139		124
ALT	12-78 U/L	57		58
T. Bili	0.2-1.3 mg/dL	9		10
Mg	1.6 – 2.6 mg/dL	1.4		
Phos	2.5-4.9 mg/dL			
TG	0-150 mg/dL	3521		
Anion gap	10-14 mMol/L	11		

Assessment:

1. Acute alcohol hepatitis: gastroenterologist consult

2. Alcoholism: initiate alcohol withdrawal protocol

3. Mixed dyslipidemia with high triglycerides: unable to treat with fenofibrate, gemfibrozil, or statins secondary to liver issues. Consult endocrinologist

4. Dehydration and hyponatremia: gentle IV normal saline, check TSH level

5. Anxiety/depression: continue Lexapro

6. Elevated serum creatinine: IV normal saline

7. Hypoalbuminemia: likely due to liver disease

8. Thrombocytopenia: likely due to liver disease

Medications administered:

- Librium: sedative
- Lexapro: anti-depressant
- MVI, Folic acid, Thiamine: part of alcohol withdrawal protocol
- Carafate: anti-ulcer
- NS @ 100 ml/hr

Discussion:

The patient has hyponatremia with decreased fluid volume related to vomiting and poor intake prior to admission. Pt was started on IV Fluids: normal saline @ 100 mls/hr to replete fluid and sodium chloride. By day two patient labs were already significantly improved. Once the EGD was completed gastritis was identified.

Case Study 2

History:

RK is a 74 year old male. For the last 4 days the patient has been experiencing nausea, vomiting, and profuse diarrhea. The patient became weak and came to the emergency department. The patient has a history of hypertension, diabetes mellitus, hypothyroidism, coronary artery disease, coronary artery bypass graft.

Labs:

Labs		3/21	3/22	3/23
Na	135-145 mMol/L	125	137	142
K	3.5 - 5 mEq/L	6.4	3.8	3.5
Cl	97-107 mEq/L	89	104	106
CO2	21-32 mEq/L	13	14	25
BUN	7-18 mg/dL	133	120	92
Creat	0.6-1.3 mg/dL	13.6	9.8	5.5
Ca	8.4-10.2 mg/dL	7.9	6.6	7
Glucose	70-99 mg/dL	411	80	121
Albumin	3.5-6g/dL	3.5	2.5	2.3

AST	15-37 U/L	10	12	18
ALT	12-78 U/L	29	18	20
T. Bili	0.2-1.3 mg/dL	0.5	0.3	0.3
Mg	1.6 – 2.6 mg/dL		1.1	1.4
Phos	2.5-4.9 mg/dL	8.8	6.4	4.8
Anion gap	10-14 mMol/L	23	19	11
Urine			Yellow/clear	
Specific gravity	1.005-1.030		1.020	
Urine pH	4.8-8		5.5	
Urine protein			Trace	
Urine glucose			negative	
Urine ketones			negative	
Urine bilirubin			negative	

Assessment:

1. Acute renal failure: secondary to diarrhea, will hydrate with IV fluids
2. Diabetic ketoacidosis: insulin drip protocol
3. Severe high anion gap metabolic acidosis: bicarbonate

4. Hypotonic, hyponatremia: IV fluids
5. Hyperlipidemia
6. Leukocytosis:
7. Gastroenteritis: recephin

Medications administered:

- Calcium gluconate: replete calcium (1g on 3/21, 1 g on 3/22)
- Pepcid: GI prophylaxis
- Rocephi: treat gastroenteritis
- Heparin: prevent blood clots
- Insulin drip: treat elevated blood sugars
- Mg Sulfate 1 g (administered 3/22): replete magnesium
- KCl 20 mEq (administered 3/22): replete potassium
- D5W + NaHCO3 @ 75 mls/hr 3/21 through 3/23
- NS @ 75 mls/hr starting 3/22

Discussion:

Patient with high anion gap acidosis caused by metabolic acidosis from diabetic ketoacidosis. The patient has hyponatremia with decreased fluid volume secondary to profuse diarrhea. The patient has developed acute renal failure due to dehydration. D5W helped replace free water. Normal saline was then started to replete sodium. Magnesium, calcium, and potassium were all repleted. Hypokalemia can occur when acidosis is treated, and when DKA is treated with insulin.

After potassium returned to normal doses of potassium were given to prevent hypokalemia.

Lab Values in Assessment of Fluid, Electrolyte and Acid-Base Balance

Albumin

3.5 - 6.0 g/dL

Indications
evaluation of chronic illness, liver disease, or nutritional status
Description
Albumin is a transport protein in the blood. It helps maintain the oncotic pressure of the blood. Albumin levels will drop if synthesis is slowed, protein intake is inadequate, or there are increased losses. Albumin has a long half life, however, so levels are not a good indicator of acute illness.
What would cause increased levels?
dehydration, hyper infusion of albumin
What would cause decreased levels?
inadequate intake, liver disease, inflammation, chronic disease, losses (fistula, hemorrhage, kidney disease, burns), over hydration, Increased catabolism, congestive heart failure

Anion gap

10-14 mMol/L

Indications

identify metabolic acidosis, identify electrolyte imbalance.

Description

Measurement of the difference between serum sodium and chloride plus bicarbonate. It is important for the number of anions and cations to be equal so that electroneutrality is maintained. Chloride and bicarbonate contribute a large portion, but the anion gap is a combinations of other anions that also contribute (phosphates, proteins, sulfates)

Anion Gap = $Na+ -- (Cl^- + HCO3)$

What would cause increased levels?

over exercise, lactic acidosis, uremia, ketoacidosis, dehydration, renal failure

What would cause decreased levels?

hypoalbuminemia, hyponatremia, hyperchloremia,

Base Excess

-2 - +2 mEq/L

Indications

identifying metabolic acidosis and alkalosis

Description

Base excess represents the amount of anions in the blood that can help buffer against changes in pH. Base excess is altered when bicarbonate levels are either high or low. If base excess is low or high it indicates a metabolic cause of acidosis or alkalosis. Negative base excess indicates metabolic acidosis.

What would cause increased levels?

metabolic alkalosis (alkali ingestion, gastric suctioning, low potassium, Cushing's disease, diuresis, diarrhea, vomiting)

What would cause decreased levels?

Metabolic acidosis (DKA, Addison's disease, Wilson's disease, renal failure, diarrhea, fistula, increased acid intake)

Bicarbonate

22-26 mEq

Indications
differentiate between metabolic and respiratory causes of pH imbalances.
Description
Bicarbonate is a base and anion that helps to neutralize acids in the blood.   Bicarbonate needs to be 20 times carbonic acid to maintain balance in the blood. Bicarbonate HCO_3^- levels can either be measured or determined using carbon dioxide levels
What would cause increased levels?
anoxia, respiratory acidosis, metabolic alkalosis
What would cause decreased levels?
hypocapnia, respiratory alkalosis, metabolic acidosis

Blood Urea Nitrogen

7-20 mg/dL

Indications
identify liver problems, renal problems, hydration status, tumor lysis; evaluate effects of drugs on liver or kidney; monitor effectiveness of hemodialysis
Description
When protein is broken down ammonia is formed. Ammonia is converted to urea in the liver and is eventually excreted in the kidneys. Blood urea

nitrogen (BUN) measures the amount of urea in the blood.

What would cause increased levels?
renal failure, CHF, kidney disease, DM, excessive protein intake, GI bleed, shock, dehydration, ketoacidosis, neoplasm, urinary tract obstruction.

What would cause decreased levels?
liver failure, over-hydration, inadequate protein intake, pregnancy

Calcium

8.4-10.2 mg/dL

Indications
identify problems with parathyroid, diseases that affect bone, effectiveness of treatments.

Description
Calcium (Ca+) is a positive ion in the body. The parathyroid gland and Vitamin D are responsible for Calcium regulation in the body. Calcium is primarily located in bone and teeth, but is also found in the blood and inside cells. Other than a major component of bone, Calcium also participates in muscle contraction. In the blood about 45% of Calcium travels in ion form, 40% is bound to proteins like albumin, 15% bound to anions like bicarbonate, lactate, etc. When albumin levels are low, Calcium levels will appear lower. Calcium has an important relationship with Phosphorus: they are inversely proportional.

What would cause increased levels?
cancers (lymphoma, leukemia, bone), acidosis, dehydration, excess calcium intake, hyperparathyroidism, pheochromocytoma,

polycythemia vera, renal transplant, sarcoidosis, vitamin D toxicity.

What would cause decreased levels?
malnutrition, cirrhosis, hypoparathyroidism, alkalosis, chronic renal failure, Magnesium deficiency, hypoalbunemia, hyperphosphatemia, malabsorption, alcoholism, osteomalacia, Vitamin D deficiency.

Chloride

97-107 mEq/L

Indications
identify different types of acidosis.

Description
Chloride (Cl^-) is an anion found in the blood. Sodium and chloride help maintain oncotic pressure and water balance in the body. Chloride is inversely related to bicarbonate levels in the blood. Chloride is a part of HCL which is utilized in the stomach to breakdown food. When red blood cells take up $CO2$ they take up chloride as well. The negative ion bicarbonate then leaves the red blood cell so that the electrical charge is maintained. Extra chloride is excreted into the urine by the kidneys.

What would cause increased levels?
dehydration, acute renal failure, Cushing's disease, hyperparathyroidism, metabolic acidosis, respiratory alkalosis.

What would cause decreased levels?
congestive heart failure, overhydration, water intoxication, burns, metabolic alkalosis, Addison's disease, salt-losing nephritis, excessive sweating, diarrhea, vomiting, fistula.

CO2

21-32 mEq/L

Indications
evaluate acid/base disturbances, and compensation
Description
CO_2 is a measure of all forms of carbon dioxide:
PCO_2 (dissolved CO_2) HCO_3, and H_2CO_3.
Carbonic acid and CO_2 are a very small portion of
this. Total CO_2 mostly reflects HCO_3
concentration.
What would cause increased levels?
metabolic alkalosis, respiratory acidosis,
tuberculosis, pneumonia, asthma attack, respiratory
depression,
What would cause decreased levels?
metabolic acidosis, respiratory acidosis, starvation,
diarrhea, dehydration, renal failure, diabetic
ketoacidosis

Creatinine

0.5-1.2 mg/dL

Indications
identify muscular disorders or renal disease.
Description
Creatinine is a byproduct of creatine metabolism, and it
is excreted in the kidneys. Creatinine is created in
proportion to muscle mass and usually stays stable.
What would cause increased levels?

gigantism, dehydration, shock, renal disease, rhabdomyolysis, acromegaly, CHF, hyperparathyroidism
What would cause decreased levels?
loss of muscle mass, inadequate protein intake, pregnancy, liver disease, muscular dystrophy

Hematocrit

Male: 41 - 50%
Female: 36 - 44%

Indications
identify anemia, bleeding, bleeding disorder, fluid imbalances.
Description
Hematocrit is the percentage of the blood that is made up of packed red blood cells. A hematocrit level of 40% indicates that there are 40 mL packed red blood cells in 100mL of blood.
What would cause increased levels?
erythrocytosis, polycythemia, shock, dehydration
What would cause decreased levels?
anemia, blood loss, bone marrow hyperplasia, severe burns

Lactic Acid

0.3 -2.6 mMol/L

Indications
determine cause of acidosis, evaluate tissue oxygenation
Description

Lactate is a byproduct of carbohydrate metabolism. Lactate is broken down by the liver. During intense exercise pyruvate is converted to lactate to provide a little extra energy when there is not enough oxygen present. If the liver doesn't properly breakdown lactate that can lead to increased levels.

What would cause increased levels?
DM, heart failure, hemorrhage, excess alcohol consumption, lactic acidosis, pulmonary embolism, reye's syndrome, shock, strenuous exercise.

What would cause decreased levels?
N/A

Magnesium

1.6 – 2.6 mg/dL

Indications
monitor renal failure, chronic alcoholism, monitor cardiac arrhythmias,

Description
Magnesium is a cation necessary for protein synthesis, nucleic acid synthesis, muscle contraction, ADP (adenosine diphosphate) use, nerve impulse conduction, and blood clotting. Magnesium affects the absorption of sodium, calcium, phosphorus, potassium.

What would cause increased levels?
Addison's disease, adrenocorticol insufficiency, dehydration, diabetic acidosis, hypothyroidism, SLE, multiple myeloma, overuse of antacids, renal insufficiency, tissue trauma

What would cause decreased levels?
alcoholism, diabetic acidosis, glomerulonephritis, hemodialysis, hypercalcemia, hypoparathyroidism,

inadequate Mg intake, malabsorption, pancreatitis, pregnancy, diarrhea

Osmolality

261 – 280 mOsm/kg

Indications
monitor electrolyte balance and acid-base balance, monitor hydration, evaluate function of antidiuretic hormone.
Description
Osmolality is a measure of the particles in solution. The size, shape, and charge of the particles do not impact the osmolality
What would cause increased levels?
dehydration, azotemia, hypercalcemia, diabetic ketoacidosis, hypernatremia, diabetes insipidus
What would cause decreased levels?
adrenocorticoid insufficiency, hyponatremia, syndrome of inappropriate antidiuretic hormone

Oxygen Saturation SaO2

95 - 100%

Indications
as part of the ABG to determine respiratory status
Description
Oxygen is transported in the blood in two ways. Oxygen dissolved in blood plasma (pO2) and oxygen bound to hemoglobin (SaO2). About 97% of oxygen is bound to hemoglobin while 3% is dissolved in plasma. There is a relationship between saturation and partial pressure referred to

the oxyhemoglobin dissociation curve. SaO2 of about 90% is associated with PO2 of about 60 mmHg.

Partial Pressure of CO2

35 - 45 mmHg

Indications
part of the ABG reflects the amount of CO2 dissolved in the blood
Description
pCO2 is an indirect measure of gas exchange within the lungs.
What would cause increased levels?
CO2 retention: pulmonary edema, COPD
What would cause decreased levels?
hyperventilation, hypoxia, anxiety, pregnancy, pulmonary embolism

Partial Pressure of O2

80 - 100 mmHg

Indications
part of an ABG to determine respiratory status

Description
Oxygen is transported in the blood in two ways. Oxygen dissolved in blood plasma (pO2) and oxygen bound to hemoglobin (SaO2). About 97% of oxygen is bound to hemoglobin while 3% is dissolved in plasma. There is a relationship between saturation and partial pressure referred to the oxyhemoglobin dissociation curve. SaO2 of about 90% is associated with PO2 of about 60 mmHg.

What would cause increased levels?
↑ O2 in inhaled air, polycythemia

What would cause decreased levels?
↓O2 in inhaled air, anemia, cardiac decompensation, COPD, restrictive pulmonary disease, hypoventilation

pH (partial pressure of Hydrogen ion)

7.35 - 7.45

Indications
identify alterations in acid/base balance

Description

reflects the amount of free H+ ions in the body

What would cause increased levels?
Metabolic alkalosis - suctioning, potassium depletion, diarrhea, vomiting
Respiratory alkalosis - stimulation of the respiratory center, hyperventilation, fever

What would cause decreased levels?
Metabolic acidosis- DKA, decreased excretion of H+, increased acid intake
Respiratory acidosis - asthma, bronchoconstriction, emphysema, pneumonia

Phosphorus

3.0-4.5 mg/dL

Indications
diagnosing hyperparathyroidism, evaluation of renal failure

Description
Phosphorus is a major intracellular anion playing a vital role in cellular metabolism. it makes up the phospholipid bilayer of the cell membrane, and is crucial in the formation of bones and teeth. Calcium and phosphorus share an inverse relationship

What would cause increased levels?
excess vitamin D, DKA, lactic acidosis, renal failure (excreted by kidneys), pulmonary embolism, respiratory acidosis, hypocalcemia, acromegaly

What would cause decreased levels?

hyperalimentation, hyperinsulinism,
hyperparathyroidism, hypokalemia, hypercalcemia,
alkalosis, vomiting and diarrhea, malnutrition,
osteomalacia

Potassium

3.5 - 5.5 mEq/L

Indications
evaluate electrolyte imbalances, useful in evaluating
cardiac arrhythmias, useful when patient is
receiving diuretic therapy, useful with acidotic
patients

Description
potassium is the most abundant intracellular cation
and plays a vital role in the transmission of
electrical impulses in cardiac and skeletal muscle.
It plays a role in acid base equilibrium. In states of
acidosis hydrogen with enter the cell as this happens
it will force potassium out of the cell, a 0.1 decrease
in pH will cause a 0.5 increase in K+.

What would cause increased levels?
acidosis, renal failure, diet, dialysis, burns,
Addison's disease, ketoacidosis, trauma,
hyperventilation, uremia

What would cause decreased levels?
CHF, alkalosis, hyperaldosteronism, toxic shock
syndrome, malabsorbtion, excess insulin, Cushing's

Sodium (serum)

135-145 mEq/L

Indications
the sodium ion is mostly found in the serum (extracellular) the test helps to evaluate total body sodium stores

Description
Sodium (Na) is the most abundant cation in extracellular fluid. Sodium aids in osmotic pressure, renal retention and excretion of water, acid-base balance, regulation of other cations and anions in the body, plays a role in blood pressure regulation, and stimulation of neuromuscular reactions. Generally speaking elevated sodium levels are often due to relative deficit of free water.

What would cause increased levels?
Cushing's disease, dehydration, burn injury, azotemia (elevated nitrogen), vomiting, lactic acidosis, fever, excessive iv fluids containing saline, diarrhea, diabetes,

What would cause decreased levels?
CHF, cystic fibrosis, diuretic use, metabolic acidosis, Addison's disease, nephrotic syndrome, excessive ADH, liver failure

Urine osmolality

50-1200 mOsm/L; l
Normal 24 hour urine osmolality: 300-900 mOsm/L

Indications
monitor electrolyte balance and acid-base balance, monitor hydration, evaluate function of antidiuretic hormone.

Description
Concentration is based on waste products of protein metabolism: urea, creatinine, uric acid

What would cause increased levels?
fluid volume deficit
SIADH: urine osmolality is inappropriately high, given the serum osmolality

What would cause decreased levels?
fluid volume excess
diabetes insipidus

Urine sodium

50-130 mEq/L

Indications
identify cause of kidney stone, identify renal disease, identify endocrine disorder, identify malabsorbtion

Description
urine sodium is affected most directly by intake. If intake increased, the body excretes excess sodium via the urine. Kidney disease can decrease the bodies ability to excrete excess sodium.

What would cause increased levels?

alkalosis, diuretic, adrenal failure, renal tubular acidosis, diabetes, excess sodium intake

What would cause decreased levels?
inadequate sodium intake, diarrhea, congestive heart failure, excessive sweating, sodium retention, prerenal azotemia

Urine specific gravity

1.001 - 1.020

Indications
identify fluid and electrolyte imbalances

Description
specific gravity is a comparison of the weight of a fluid compared to the weight of water. Specific gravity is affected by both the weight and amount of particles. Osmolality is not affected by the size, just the number of particles. Glucose and protein are large molecules that will have a greater impact on specific gravity in the urine more than smaller particles.

What would cause increased levels?
fluid volume deficit
SIADH: urine osmolality is inappropriately high, given the serum osmolality

What would cause decreased levels?
fluid volume excess
diabetes insipidus

Osmolality	Specific gravity
350 mOsm/kg	1.010
7200 mOsm/kg	1.020
1050 mOsm/kg	1.030
1400 mOsm/L	1.040

Urine ph

4.8-8

Indications
identify alterations in acid/base balance

Description
Kidneys help balance pH in the blood by eliminating hydrogen ions. During acidosis the urine pH should decrease. If the pH is high, this indicates a problem within the kidneys (renal tubular acidosis). During metabolic alkalosis the pH should be high. If it is low this may indicate volume depletion. During volume depletion the body retains sodium in the form of Sodium Bicarbonate.

What would cause increased levels?
Metabolic alkalosis - suctioning, diarrhea, vomiting
Respiratory alkalosis - stimulation of the respiratory center, hyperventilation, fever

What would cause decreased levels?
Metabolic acidosis- DKA, increased acid intake
Respiratory acidosis - asthma, bronchoconstriction, emphysema, pneumonia

NCLEX Fluid and Electrolyte Questions

Management of Care

1. A nurse is caring for a patient who has developed severe hyponatremia and is confused. The nurse needs help with caring for the patient's needs while keeping the patient safe without using restraints. Which of the following best demonstrates that the nurse is protecting the privacy of this patient?
   a. Keeping the patient's secrets when she tells the nurse something important
   b. Discussing the patient's condition with other staff to determine the best course of action
   c. Not telling the family about the patient's behavior because it would embarrass her
   d. Placing the patient in a room near the nurse's station

D – When a patient is being uncooperative or dangerous, restraints may be necessary to keep the patient confined. The nurse should try to avoid using restraints if at all possible by coming up with alternative solutions when the patient is uncooperative. In this case, the nurse could protect the patient's privacy and dignity by placing her in a room near the nurse's station where the staff can monitor her more closely.

2. A patient is recovering from surgery and has been placed in the post-anesthesia care unit for monitoring. The patient is going to be discharged to extended care in one of the hospital units. Which condition would require that the nurse monitor the patient further before discharging him?

a. The patient is bleeding
b. The patient has sutures on his surgical wound
c. The patient's blood pressure is 110/80 mmHg
d. The patient needs pain medication

A – Transfer from the recovery room to the unit where the patient will stay requires that the patient be in a state of relatively stable health that does not require constant monitoring. If a patient is actively bleeding after surgery, he is not stable enough to be moved to the floor and must remain in the recovery room until the bleeding is under control.

3. A nurse is caring for a patient who requires intravenous fluids to prevent fluid and electrolyte imbalance. The nurse has developed a clinical pathway to direct care of this patient. What best describes the purpose of a clinical pathway?
a. To determine what decisions should be made in case the patient develops complications
b. To describe tasks needed to care for a patient's specific condition
c. To set up parameters for monitoring that the patient has met his goals
d. To consider how long the patient will need care from the nurse

B – A clinical pathway is a plan of patient care that describes tasks that are required for care of a patient's specific condition. The clinical pathway also outlines goals that are designed for the patient's condition. In this way, clinical pathways differ between patients because no two patients are exactly alike. The nurse can develop a clinical pathway to guide her work as she cares for the patient's specific needs.

4. A 77-year-old patient is suffering from heart failure. The nurse has given him a nursing diagnosis of Fluid Volume Excess related to heart failure as evidenced by weight gain and peripheral edema. Which of the following interventions should the nurse employ with this nursing diagnosis?

a. Monitor the patient's intake and output every 24 hours

b. Keep the patient's legs in the dependent position

c. Place the patient on a low-magnesium diet

d. Auscultate breath sounds at least every 2 hours

D – Fluid volume excess develops when the patient has excess circulating volume in the bloodstream or the body is retaining enough fluid that the excess is in the tissues outside of circulation. It may be manifested by such signs or symptoms as swelling, "wet" breath sounds, and weight gain. Nursing interventions include reducing edema, checking breath sounds regularly for changes, and monitoring intake and output at least every 4 hours.

5. A nurse is working with a patient who has an electrolyte imbalance due to inflammatory bowel disease. Which of the following information should the nurse provide to the patient about his food and fluid intake?
a. In order to avoid constipation, the patient should take a stool softener
b. The patient is at increased risk of hemorrhoids, which can be avoided by eating more fiber
c. The patient may be more likely to feel weak and dizzy if he develops dehydration
d. In order to stay hydrated, the patient should drink 16 oz. of fluid for every pound of body weight daily

C – A patient with inflammatory bowel disease is at increased risk of dehydration because of excess diarrhea as a result of the condition. The diarrhea causes fluid loss and electrolyte imbalance when it is not managed. The patient may become weak and dizzy if he becomes dehydrated, which puts him at further risk of injury because of his condition.

6. Following a patient's first session of hemodialysis, the nurse is providing information to the patient and his family about his care at home. Which information should the patient be aware of that will prevent damage to the hemodialysis fistula site?
a. Do not lift anything heavy with the arm that has the hemodialysis access site
b. Inject a solution of heparin and normal saline into the site daily to prevent clotting
c. Wear a medical alert bracelet on the affected arm to notify caregivers of the access site
d. Do not shower and keep the arm covered while bathing as long as the fistula is in place

A – A patient who requires hemodialysis may have a fistula placed in the arm, which acts as an access site for the procedure. The patient must take care of the arm with the access site to avoid displacing the fistula so it can continue to be used long term for dialysis. The patient should be taught to avoid lifting heavy items with the affected arm and to avoid wearing watches or anything constricting on the arm with the fistula.

7. An interdisciplinary team works on the medical-surgical unit of the hospital to provide comprehensive care for their complex group of patients. Which best describes the role of the dietitian on the team in managing fluid and electrolyte balance?

a. Teaching patients about how to control fluid intake while in the hospital

b. Helping patients choose foods from their menus that provide enough nutrition and fluids

c. Weighing patients daily and reporting the results to the physicians

d. Checking blood glucose levels of patients to determine if they have blood sugar instability

B – The dietitian on the interdisciplinary team is able to provide guidance and care related to food and fluid intakes of patients. This typically means teaching patients about appropriate foods and dietary practices that are healthy. The dietitian may help some patients with making appropriate choices from their menus so that they get enough nutrients in their diets.

8. A patient is suffering from fluid overload due to a history of severe liver disease. Which of the following interventions would be the highest priority for this patient?
a. Weigh the patient daily
b. Elevate the lower extremities to reduce edema
c. Monitor for heart arrhythmias and the presence of crackles on auscultation
d. Check skin regularly for signs of skin breakdown

C – Fluid overload can develop as a result of various types of disease processes; it can lead to edema, weight gain, and electrolyte imbalance. To avoid complications of fluid overload, the nurse should listen to the patient's heart rate to determine if excess fluid has caused heart arrhythmias; the nurse should also listen to the patient's breath sounds for signs of breathing difficulties because of increased fluid.

Safety and Infection Control

9. A nurse is caring for a patient who is recovering from surgery and she must contact the healthcare provider for orders for IV fluids. Which of the following must the nurse consider when taking an order over the phone from a physician?

a. Another nurse should listen to the call to verify that the order is correct

b. The nurse should read the order back to the physician and document this information in the patient's chart

c. The nurse should ask the provider to come to the unit to sign the order within the next hour

d. The nurse should never take orders over the phone; it is not allowed by law

B – Telephone orders have the potential for mistakes, as the provider may try to relay information over the phone that can be misheard or written down incorrectly. Because of this, the nurse should avoid trying to take telephone orders if possible. If it is unavoidable, the nurse should take a telephone order and then read the information back to the physician to ensure it is correct. The read back must be documented in the patient's chart.

10. A 63-year-old patient with cirrhosis is telling the nurse about his extreme fatigue that he must work around every day. Which intervention related to the patient's food and fluid intake should the nurse suggest that would best help in this situation?

a. Decrease carbohydrate intake and focus on increasing fats and protein in the diet
b. Increase intake of vitamin D to provide a source of energy
c. Increase fluid intake and intake of foods that contain water or juice
d. Decrease fiber intake and add more salt to foods when cooking

C – Fatigue is a common side effect that can cause difficulty for the patient who must continue to work while feeling exhausted because of symptoms. The patient who is fatigued may make some dietary changes that can help to improve symptoms. The patient should be encouraged to increase carbohydrate intake for energy and to drink more fluids or eat foods that contain water or juice.

Health Promotion and Maintenance

11. A nurse in the newborn nursery is caring for a baby who was born 3 days ago. The infant weight 6 lbs., 12 oz. at birth. After the daily weight, the nurse notes that the infant now weighs 5 lbs., 8 oz. Which action of the nurse is most appropriate?
    a. Continue to monitor the infant's normal weight loss after birth
    b. Encourage the mother to breastfeed the infant and then weigh him again
    c. Check the infant's glucose level
    d. Notify the physician about the baby's condition

D – It is normal for a newborn infant to lose some body weight after birth; most healthcare providers consider a loss of up to 7 percent of original body weight to be within normal limits. Loss of more than this, such as in this situation, requires contacting the healthcare provider for further orders. The nurse should not try to make the infant eat first; at this point, the physician needs to know to manage the patient's weight.

12. A 19-year-old college student is seen in the university health clinic for symptoms of dehydration and weight loss. The patient is a member of the school's track team and spends several hours a day training. Which information should the nurse give to this patient to prevent dehydration associated with excessive exercise?

a. Establish a baseline body weight by weighing every week to determine fluid needs

b. Drink fluids starting several hours before exercise begins

c. Avoid electrolyte replacement beverages when exercising and drink only water

d. Remember that fluid replacement after exercise cannot fully replace that which was lost with activity

B – A person who exercises a great amount, such as with a student athlete, may be at risk of dehydration and electrolyte imbalance from water loss through sweat and respiration. The nurse should counsel the patient to drink electrolyte replacement beverages or water and to drink fluids throughout the entire period: before, during, and after exercising.

13. An 86-year-old male patient is transferred from the long-term care facility where he lives to the hospital for treatment after falling in the hallway. The staff tell the nurse that he normally is not a fall risk and has been healthy and active, with little to no cognitive impairments. Upon admission, the patient's laboratory workup indicates that he is severely dehydrated. Which of the following manifestations of dehydration would more likely develop in an older adult? Select all that apply.
   a. Rapid breathing rate
   b. Confusion
   c. Convulsions
   d. Diarrhea
   e. Insomnia

A, B, C – Dehydration may be manifested slightly differently among elderly patients when compared to younger adults. An older adult patient may have standard symptoms of dehydration, including rapid respiratory rate and poor skin turgor, but the elderly patient may also suffer from other effects as well, such as confusion or convulsions.

14. An older adult has been diagnosed with elderly failure to thrive based on his increased weight loss, poor nutrition, and dehydration. Which medical condition has also been associated with adult failure to thrive? Select all that apply.
a. Substance abuse
b. Skin cancer
c. Renal failure
d. Stroke
e. Arthritis

A, C, D, E – Adult failure to thrive is a condition characterized by poor nutrition, poor growth, and increased instances of illness, such as dehydration or poor immune system function. Adult failure to thrive is associated with a number of medical conditions that can lead to poor health of the adult patient, including such conditions as substance abuse, renal failure, stroke, or arthritis.

Psychosocial Integrity

15. After being admitted as an inpatient for treatment of substance abuse, a patient begins to experience delirium tremens. He is confused and disoriented and is demonstrating tachycardia, sweating, and tremor. Which nursing intervention is most appropriate for management of delirium tremens?
    a. Administer pain medications to promote patient comfort
    b. Monitor the patient's cardiac status with a hemodynamic monitor
    c. Restrict fluid intake until the patient demonstrates appropriate swallowing ability
    d. Elevate the feet to promote venous return

B – Delirium tremens is a condition that develops in response to withdrawal from alcohol. It most commonly occurs with alcohol addiction, when the body has become accustomed to alcohol intake. The patient may have increased sweating, shakiness, and tachycardia, and may suffer from hallucinations. The nurse should monitor the patient's heart rate and provide a calm environment to help him through this difficult transition.

16. A 56-year-old patient is struggling with a diagnosis of kidney disease. The patient says to the nurse, "I don't think I can handle this. How can I watch everything I eat and drink and then still go to dialysis?" The nurse can best help the patient with recognizing coping mechanisms by responding:

a. "You may still be able to have hemodialysis at home; that would make it easier for you."

b. "You do not need to watch what you eat or drink if you are having dialysis anyway."

c. "Tell me about what makes you feel better when you are in an unfamiliar situation."

d. "You feel conflicted about your dialysis treatments."

C – A diagnosis of a chronic disease such as kidney failure that requires dialysis can be a lot of information for a patient to accept. The patient may have difficulties with coping with the diagnosis and may feel confused and upset. The nurse can help the patient to recognize what coping mechanisms have worked in the past and to utilize those familiar mechanisms to help him try to accept this situation.

17. A nurse is caring for a postpartum patient who is Vietnamese and speaks little English. Because of complications with delivery, the mother experienced a larger amount of blood loss, and the physician has ordered for an increase in IV fluids as well as pushing oral intake of fluids. The nurse brings the mother a pitcher of ice water and the patient becomes visibly upset. Which response from the nurse is most appropriate?

a. "You need to drink water so you will not become dehydrated."

b. "Would you feel better having something different to drink?"

c. "Is there something wrong that you do not like water?"

d. "Are you having any pain?"

B – The nurse in this situation should recognize that the patient most likely has cultural factors that she wants to adhere to after delivery. The patient may have specific beliefs about drinking cold fluids and has become upset. The nurse should recognize that some cultural methods are different from her own and try to find a solution by asking the patient about what she would like to drink.

Basic Care and Comfort

18. A 67-year-old patient is at an appointment at the healthcare clinic and is visiting with the nurse in the healthcare office. The patient's spouse tells the nurse that the patient does not always respond when she talks to him and he doesn't participate in family activities as much anymore. Which step should the nurse perform first?

a. Check inside the patient's ear for occlusion

b. Stand behind the patient and perform the whispered voice test

c. Ask the patient and his spouse to fill out a hearing loss questionnaire

d. Perform a pure-tone audiometry test in the office

A – The risk of hearing loss increases as an adult grows older, and the nurse may have several tests that she can perform that could determine whether the patient is suffering from hearing loss. Without further information, the first step of the nurse is to look inside the patient's ears to determine if there is a physical occlusion present that is contributing to the hearing loss.

19. A 56-year-old patient has been hospitalized for acute renal failure. During her shift, the nurse notes that the patient's urine output has dropped to 5 mL/hour, despite a continuous infusion of IV fluids at a rate of 150 mL/hr. If left uncorrected, which complication would the nurse most likely expect to see?
a. Metabolic alkalosis
b. Decreased BUN and creatinine levels
c. Diarrhea and poor skin turgor
d. Pulmonary edema

D – When measuring urine output for a hospitalized patient, the typical standard outcome that indicates normal output is 30 mL/hr. A patient with urine output of 5 mL/hr most likely has a condition that is preventing the body from making urine or from excreting it properly. If not corrected, the patient may develop other complications, including pulmonary edema and metabolic acidosis.

20. Which of the following changes in elimination would most likely occur in a patient who is unable to get out of bed and is immobile? Select all that apply.
a. Positive nitrogen balance
b. Urinary stasis
c. Increased risk of kidney stones
d. Diarrhea
e. Urinary tract infections

B, C, E – Immobility can cause a number of
physical changes in a patient; immobility reduces
blood flow, which can affect multiple body systems.
The immobile patient is at higher risk of skin
breakdown, blood clots, urinary stasis, kidney
stones, and urinary tract infections.

21. A 66-year-old patient has become dehydrated after being outside in the sun for too long. The patient complains of feeling dizzy and lightheaded. Which of the following nursing diagnoses is most appropriate in this situation?
a. Ineffective Health Maintenance
b. Imbalanced Nutrition: Less than Body Requirements
c. Risk for Electrolyte Imbalance
d. Impaired Urinary Elimination

C – A patient who is dehydrated is at risk of electrolyte imbalance due to the loss of fluid from the body. The amount of electrolytes may become more concentrated in the body when there is less fluid within circulation. The patient may experience a number of negative effects, including nausea, dizziness, and confusion.

22. A 15-year-old patient is being treated at the hospital for severe diarrhea following a bacterial infection. Which of the following interventions should the nurse use that would best prevent this patient from developing severe dehydration?
a. Help the patient to drink plenty of water
b. Begin an infusion of insulin IV
c. Assist the patient with taking in plenty of broth, fruit juice, and vegetable soup
d. Administer a dose of bismuth subsalicylate (Pepto Bismol®) and repeat as needed

C – Severe diarrhea can lead to significant dehydration if the condition is not well managed. Children and older adults are at higher risk of complications from dehydration. In this case, the patient should be encouraged to drink fluids such as broth and fruit juice, which contain electrolytes in addition to fluid and can provide some replacement.

Pharmacological and Parenteral Therapies

23. Which of the following fluids would be considered a type of crystalloid solution?
    a. Hartmann's solution
    b. 6% hydroxyethyl starch
    c. Albumin
    d. 4% succinylated gelatin

A – Crystalloid solutions are clear fluids that can be administered intravenously to correct fluid balance. Crystalloids are easily accessible and are usually cheaper when compared to colloid solutions. Hartmann's solution, also called compound sodium lactate, is an example of a crystalloid solution.

24. A nurse is providing post-operative care for a patient who is recovering from bowel surgery. The patient had excess bleeding during the procedure and the physician has ordered a colloid solution to replete intravascular volume. In addition to volume expansion, what best describes an advantage of using colloid solutions over crystalloids?
a. Colloids are less likely to cause antibody reactions
b. Colloids are cheaper to administer when compared to crystalloids
c. Colloids produce less edema and require smaller volumes
d. Colloids reduce the risk of renal toxicity when administered

C – When providing intravenous fluids, the provider has a choice of using colloid or crystalloid solutions. Generally, crystalloids are cheaper and easier to access, while colloids do not require as large of amounts to achieve the same effects and they produce less edema. Albumin is an example of a colloid solution.

25. A patient who has been severely burned in an accident is brought to the emergency department. The physician orders a regimen to begin fluid resuscitation. Which type of fluid would the nurse most likely use as part of fluid resuscitation following a burn injury?
a. 0.9% Normal saline
b. Lactated Ringer's solution
c. D10W
d. D5 ½ NS with KCl

B – When a patient is severely burned, he requires a significant amount of fluid replacement in the first 24 hours, known as fluid resuscitation. Lactated Ringer's solution is typically the fluid of choice because it is easy to access, which is important because the patient will need a lot of fluid. Lactated Ringer's is an isotonic solution that contains a small amount of electrolytes.

26. In which situation would the administration of a loop diuretic (Lasix®) be most appropriate?
   a. Anuria
   b. Pulmonary edema
   c. Hyponatremia
   d. Cirrhosis

B – Lasix is a loop diuretic that is used to release excess salt into the urine, instead of it being reabsorbed into the bloodstream. It is most commonly used in conditions of excess fluid, such as pulmonary edema, heart failure, or nephrotic syndrome.

27. A 67-year-old patient is being seen following an arm fracture. The patient was diagnosed with osteoporosis last year and has been making lifestyle changes to manage the condition. The physician now wants to start the patient on medication to control the disease. Which type of medication would most likely be prescribed to prevent the breakdown of bone tissue in the body?
a. Biological response modifiers
b. Glucocorticoids
c. Cholinergics
d. Biphosphonates

D – Biphosphonates are drugs used for the treatment of osteoporosis. They work by preventing the breakdown of bone tissue in the body that leads to bone loss. Examples of biphosphonates include Fosamax and Boniva.

28. A patient with a history of alcoholism is in the hospital following an illness. The patient is significantly malnourished and the physician has ordered TPN for replacement of electrolytes. After starting on TPN, the patient develops refeeding syndrome. Which of the following symptoms of abnormal brain function would the nurse expect to see?
a. Hydrocephalus
b. Meningitis
c. Wernicke's encephalopathy
d. Intracerebral hemorrhage

C – A patient who is severely malnourished may develop refeeding syndrome in response to suddenly being administered adequate nourishment through TPN. Refeeding syndrome causes electrolyte imbalance, including an imbalance of thiamine. This leads to symptoms of Wernicke's encephalopathy, which causes confusion and balance problems.

29. A patient is brought into the emergency department after suffering from third degree burns in an explosion. The patient has burns on approximately 40 percent of his body. The nurse weighs the patient and notes that he weighs 170 lbs. Calculate the rate of IV fluid this patient must receive in the first 24 hours using the Parkland formula.

a. 4 L
b. 8 L
c. 12 L
d. 16 L

C – The Parkland formula is a method of calculating the amount of fluid needed for fluid resuscitation after a burn injury. To use the Parkland formula, the nurse must know the weight of the patient in kg and the approximate size of the burn. To determine the amount, the nurse multiplies the percent of body surface area burned by the patient's weight in kg and multiplies that outcome by 4mL. The first half of the result should be given in the first 8 hours, with the second half of the result given in the following 16 hours.

30. A patient with diabetes insipidus must start taking vasopressin. Which information from the nurse is correct when providing teaching about this medication?

a. Vasopressin is taken as an oral tablet or in syrup form

b. The patient will need to increase his or her fluid intake while on this medication

c. The physician may order a routine ECG while the patient is taking vasopressin

d. Vasopressin can cause severe hypomagnesemia as a potential side effect

C – Vasopressin is a synthetic form of anti-diuretic hormone; it works by helping the body reabsorb water through the kidneys and by improving blood pressure. When a patient must take this medication, the nurse should let him or her know that some tests are required while the patient is taking the drug. For example, the patient may need routine ECG testing to monitor heart function while on this drug.

31. A 67-year-old patient with renal dysfunction has received a prescription for hydrochlorothiazide tablets. Which condition is considered a contraindication for using this drug?
a. Anuria
b. Cirrhosis
c. Heart failure
d. Hypothyroidism

A – Hydrochlorothiazide is a type of thiazide diuretic that prevents the body from absorbing too much salt in the bloodstream. The drug prevents fluid buildup and edema from fluid retention. It is most often used for heart failure, cirrhosis, and kidney failure, but it should not be used in conditions in which the patient does not make urine.

Reduction of Risk Potential

32. The process of the breakdown of large molecules into small ones, such as when proteins are broken down into amino acids, is known as:
a. anabolism
b. hydrolysis.
c. catabolism.
d. dehydration synthesis.

C – Catabolism is the process of breaking down some large molecules into smaller ones that the body can use. For example, when a person ingests foods that contain protein, the body breaks these down through catabolism into amino acids.

33. Following a case of acute pancreatitis, a patient's health continues to decline until he develops systemic inflammatory response syndrome (SIRS). What vital sign results would the nurse expect to see in this condition?
a. Respiratory rate less than 8/min
b. Temperature greater than 100.4°F
c. Heart rate greater than 120 bpm
d. Blood pressure greater than 140/90 mmHg

B –Systemic inflammatory response syndrome (SIRS) is a condition in which the body is progressing into a state of sepsis. The patient with SIRS develops widespread inflammation, elevated temperature, and tachycardia. If the patient has a bacterial infection that is causing the widespread inflammation, he or she is said to have sepsis.

34. A patient is seen in the primary care clinic after having excess vomiting for 3 days. The physician orders a CBC and metabolic panel to assess for underlying illness. Which of the following lab results would most likely appear after consistent vomiting?
a.   Increased hematocrit
b.   Decreased AST/ALT
c.   Increased sodium
d.   Decreased creatinine

A – Hematocrit describes the percentage of red blood cells in the blood. When a patient has excessive vomiting over a period of time, he or she loses intravascular volume with dehydration. The decreased volume of fluid causes an increase in the concentration of red blood cells and an increase in hematocrit.

35. Which laboratory result best indicates a normal amount of serum chloride?
a. 1.1-3.8 mEq/L
b. 10-18 mEq/L
c. 22.5-30 mEq/L
d. 95-105 mEq/L

D – Chloride is a type of electrolyte in the bloodstream that may be measured with an electrolyte panel blood test to check for abnormalities or electrolyte imbalance. The normal amount of serum chloride is between 95 and 105 mEq/L.

36. A patient who is in liver failure is hospitalized for management of symptoms. The physician has ordered an arterial blood gas, which demonstrates that the patient is in a state of metabolic acidosis. What symptoms would the nurse most likely see in this case?
a. Hypotension
b. Peripheral edema
c. Rapid respiratory rate
d. Exophthalmos

C – Metabolic acidosis is a state in which there is too much acid in the body fluids. It most often results in symptoms associated with its cause, but it can also lead to a rapid respiratory rate, confusion, and lethargy.

37. A 56-year-old patient is suffering from interstitial nephritis and is seen in the hospital for care. The patient's creatinine levels are elevated and he has poor skin turgor and dry mucous membranes upon exam. As part of patient care, the nurse ensures that the patient does not receive any nephrotoxic medications that would worsen his condition. Which medication should be avoided?

a. Gentamicin
b. Abilify
c. Combivir
d. Amantadine

A – Nephrotoxic medications are those that can cause damage to the kidneys. When a patient is at risk, nephrotoxic drugs could cause such damage that a patient goes into a state of acute renal failure. Some antibiotics are nephrotoxic drugs and should be used very carefully in at-risk patients. An example of a nephrotoxic drug that is an antibiotic is gentamicin.

38. A patient has a nasogastric tube placed after developing a paralytic ileus following surgery. The nurse maintains the NG tube and performs interventions to ensure adequate hydration for the patient. Which intervention is most closely associated with assessment of fluid intake and output in a patient with an NG tube?

a. Assessing daily for peripheral edema
b. Considering fluid losses from the patient's perspiration, hyperventilation, and wound drainage
c. Monitoring for cognitive changes in the patient's sensory level system
d. Determining whether the patient has abdominal pain

B – Placement of a nasogastric tube often means that the patient is unable to take in food and fluids by mouth. When this occurs, the patient is at high risk of fluid loss because of decreased intake. The nurse must ensure that the patient takes enough fluid and should closely monitor intake and output. The nurse should also consider other potential losses of fluid, such as through respiration and wound drainage.

Physiological Adaptation

39. A recovery room nurse is caring for a patient who is recovering from anesthesia after colon surgery. The nurse is providing IV fluids of ½ NS at a rate of 150 mL/hr to the patient. In order to avoid complications associated with fluid administration, which intervention would the nurse most likely perform?
   a. Elevate the extremity that has the IV
   b. Increase the rate of the IV for the first hour and then turn it down to a very low rate
   c. Apply a pressure support sleeve to the IV bag
   d. Maintain IV administration with a fluid pump instead of gravity

D – A patient recovering from surgery can be at risk of fluid overload if the IV fluids run too fast or are not well controlled. In some recovery room environments, the patients are given IV fluids by gravity, which must be watched closely to avoid giving too much fluid at once. The nurse can reduce the risk of too high volume administration by using a fluid pump instead of administering fluid by gravity.

40. A patient with celiac disease has developed hypomagnesemia from malabsorption. Which sign or symptom would the nurse expect to see with this condition?
a. Muscle cramps and weakness
b. Respiratory depression
c. Hypotension
d. Cardiac arrest

A – Hypomagnesemia occurs when magnesium levels in the blood are lower than normal. The condition develops from such illnesses as malabsorption syndromes, alcoholism, or chronic diarrhea. A patient with hypomagnesemia will most likely demonstrate muscle cramps, weakness, and fatigue.

41. A 67-year-old patient has been suffering from alcohol abuse and has developed severe hypokalemia with a potassium level of 2.9 mEq/L. An hour after admission to the hospital, the patient develops a cardiac dysrhythmia because of his potassium levels. The rhythm on the monitor shows pulseless electrical activity (PEA). Which action should the nurse perform next?

a. Start CPR by using chest compressions at a rate of 100 per minute
b. Charge the defibrillator to administer a shock
c. Provide 2 rescue breaths and reassess the heart rhythm
d. Administer adenosine and place the patient in the recovery position

A – When a patient enters cardiac arrest and has a rhythm of PEA on the monitor, the provider must continue to perform chest compressions to support blood flow. PEA does not produce electrical activity and will not respond to a shock from an AED.

42. A 70-year-old patient with hypovolemia has been given the nursing diagnosis of Altered Tissue Perfusion by the nurse. Which outcome listed would be most appropriate as a treatment goal for this patient?
a. Urine output of at least 20 mL/hr
b. Bounding peripheral pulses
c. Cool extremities with no cyanosis
d. Blood pressure within the normal range for the patient

D – A patient with altered tissue perfusion most likely has a condition in which he does not have enough blood flow to perfuse the organs and peripheral extremities. The nurse should focus her interventions on improving blood flow to prevent tissue ischemia. Signs of improved tissue perfusion include warm skin, palpable pulses, and blood pressure within normal limits for the patient.

43. A patient is recovering from abdominal surgery when he develops sudden and profuse bleeding from the surgical site. Which of the following signs or symptoms should the nurse check for that would indicate altered cerebral perfusion as a result of bleeding?
a. Irritability and restlessness
b. Dilated pupils
c. Headache
d. Inability to speak

A – Altered tissue perfusion from bleeding can affect the organs and tissues, including the brain. When there is not enough blood flow to the brain, the patient will develop cognitive changes. Irritability and restlessness are two cardinal signs of altered cerebral tissue perfusion associated with blood loss.

Your Free Gift!
As a way of saying thanks for your purchase, I'm offering a
free PDF download:

"63 Must Know NCLEX® Labs"

With these charts you will be able to take the 63 most
important labs with you anywhere you go!
You can download the 4 page PDF document by clicking here,
or going to NRSNG.com/labs

About the Authors

Jon Haws RN CCRN: Sick of spending hours and hours trying to find all the information you need for clinical and NCLEX® study? So was I . . . . That's why I created NRSNG.com, a community of nurses and nursing students wanting to jump start their careers.

I am a registered nurse and CCRN on a Neurovascular Intensive Care Unit at a Level I Trauma Hospital. I attended college at Brigham Young University and later received my Nursing degree from Methodist College in Peoria, IL. I also hold a Business Management degree from Touro University.

Professionally, I precept nursing students and new graduate Registered Nurses and work as a charge nurse . . . and love it!

Come visit us at NRSNG.com or check in on Facebook.com/NRSNG.

Sandra Haws MS RD CNSC: is a dietitian with one of the largest health care systems in the United States. She works with intensive care patients. She obtained her undergraduate degree from Brigham Young University and her graduate degree from Texas Woman's University. She holds advanced certifications in nutrition support management.

Visit NursingStudentBooks.com to view more books.

Made in the USA
Columbia, SC
05 August 2017